A USMLE S

MW01050718

Surgery

11th Edition

A USMLE STEP 2 REVIEW

Surgery
11th Edition

700
Questions & Answers

Written by faculty of the
Department of Surgery
University of Missouri—Columbia
School of Medicine
Columbia, Missouri

edited by
Michael H. Metzler, MD, FACS, FCCM
John W. Growdon Distinguished Associate Professor;
Chief, Divisions of General Surgery
and Surgical Critical Care;
Associate Professor of Anesthesiology

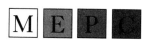

Medical Examination
Publishing Company

APPLETON & LANGE
Norwalk, Connecticut

95 96 97 98 / 10 9 8 7 6 5 4 3 2 1

Prentice Hall International (UK) Limited, *London*
Prentice Hall of Australia Pty. Limited, *Sydney*
Prentice Hall Canada, Inc., *Toronto*
Prentice Hall Hispanoamericana, S.A., *Mexico*
Prentice Hall of India Private Limited, *New Delhi*
Prentice Hall of Japan, Inc., *Tokyo*
Simon & Schuster Asia Pte. Ltd., *Singapore*
Editora Prentice Hall do Brasil Ltda., *Rio de Janeiro*
Prentice Hall, *Englewood Cliffs, New Jersey*

ISBN 0-8385-6195-0

90000

9 780838 561959

ISBN: 0-8385-6195-0
ISSN: 1080-9279

Acquisitions Editor: Jamie Mount Kircher
Production Services: Rainbow Graphics, Inc.

PRINTED IN THE UNITED STATES OF AMERICA

To our teachers, students,
colleagues, and families . . .
from whom we have learned

Contents

Contributors . . . .   *ix*
Preface . . . .   *xi*
Acknowledgment . . . .   *xiii*
References . . . .   *xv*

1. Basic Surgical Science   1
    Answers and Comments   15
    Michael H. Metzler

2. Statistics and Clinical Literature Interpretation   24
    Answers and Comments   32
    Jeffrey O. Phillips

3. Abdominal Surgery   37
    Answers and Comments   57
    Brent W. Miedema

4. Breast and Endocrine Surgery   71
    Answers and Comments   86
    Debra G. Koivunen and Paul Yazdi

5. Urologic Surgery and Transplantation   97
    Answers and Comments   111
    Stephen H. Weinstein and Michael S. Callister

6. Plastic and Reconstructive Surgery   120
    Answers and Comments   128
    Gregory H. Croll

7. Otolaryngology.................................... 134
    Answers and Comments 147
    Paul R. Cook

8. Neurology.. 153
    Answers and Comments 164
    John J. Oro and Scott R. Gibbs

9. Surgery of Trauma and Burns 168
    Answers and Comments 184
    Tina L. Palmieri and Michael H. Metzler

10. Orthopaedic Surgery.............................. 195
    Answers and Comments 212
    Barry J. Gainor and James M. Banovetz, Jr.

11. Cardiothoracic Surgery........................... 222
    Answers and Comments 236
    Richard A. Schmaltz

12. Peripheral Vascular Surgery...................... 248
    Answers and Comments 270
    W. Kirt Nichols and Michael Kikta

13. Pediatric Surgery 279
    Answers and Comments 294
    Mary Alice Helikson and Patricia Barker

14. Case Studies 304
    Answers and Comments 313

Contributors

James M. Banovetz, Jr., PhD, MD, Chief Resident, Division of Orthopaedic Surgery, University of Missouri—Columbia School of Medicine, Columbia, Missouri

Patricia Barker, MD, Senior Resident, Division of General Surgery, University of Missouri—Columbia School of Medicine, Columbia, Missouri

Michael S. Callister, MD, Resident, Urology, University of Missouri—Columbia School of Medicine, Columbia, Missouri

Paul R. Cook, MD, Assistant Professor, Division of Otolaryngology, University of Missouri—Columbia School of Medicine, Columbia, Missouri

Gregory H. Croll, MD, Assistant Professor, Division of Plastic and Reconstructive Surgery, University of Missouri—Columbia School of Medicine, Columbia, Missouri

Barry J. Gainor, MD, Professor, Division of Orthopaedic Surgery, University of Missouri—Columbia School of Medicine, Columbia, Missouri

Scott R. Gibbs, MA, MD, Senior Resident, Division of Neurological Surgery, University of Missouri—Columbia School of Medicine, Columbia, Missouri

Mary Alice Helikson, MD, Assistant Professor, Section Pediatric Surgery, University of Missouri—Columbia School of Medicine, Columbia, Missouri

Michael Kikta, MD, Vascular Fellow, Division of Vascular Surgery, University of Missouri—Columbia School of Medicine, Columbia, Missouri

Debra G. Koivunen, MD, Assistant Professor, Division of General Surgery, University of Missouri—Columbia School of Medicine, Columbia, Missouri

Michael H. Metzler, MD, FACS, FCCM, John W. Growdon Distinguished Associate Professor; Chief, Divisions of General Surgery and Surgical Critical Care; Associate Professor of Anesthesiology, University of Missouri—Columbia School of Medicine, Columbia, Missouri

Brent W. Miedema, MD, Assistant Professor, Division of General Surgery, University of Missouri—Columbia School of Medicine, Columbia, Missouri

W. Kirt Nichols, MD, Professor, Divisions of General and Vascular Surgery, University of Missouri—Columbia School of Medicine, Columbia, Missouri

John J. Oro, MD, Associate Professor and Chief, Division of Neurological Surgery, University of Missouri—Columbia School of Medicine, Columbia, Missouri

Tina L. Palmieri, MD, Critical Care and Burn Fellow, Divisions of General Surgery and Surgical Critical Care, University of Missouri—Columbia School of Medicine, Columbia, Missouri

Jeffrey O. Phillips, Pharm D., Assistant Professor, Division of Surgical Critical Care, University of Missouri—Columbia School of Medicine, Columbia, Missouri

Richard A. Schmaltz, MD, Assistant Professor, Division of Cardiothoracic Surgery, University of Missouri—Columbia School of Medicine, Columbia, Missouri

Stephen H. Weinstein, MD, Associate Professor, Division of Urology, University of Missouri—Columbia School of Medicine, Columbia, Missouri

Paul Yazdi, MD, Senior Resident, General Surgery, University of Missouri—Columbia School of Medicine, Columbia, Missouri

Preface

The multiple authorship of this 11th edition by members of the Department of Surgery, University of Missouri–Columbia, reflects the ever-increasing body of fundamental scientific and clinical knowledge which provides the basis of surgical practice. Each section author has developed questions which emphasize major concepts and pertinent information from his or her individual specialty area. Clinical presentation, mechanisms of disease processes, prevention, and principles of management are stressed in each section. A new section has been added to emphasize the importance of statistics in interpretation of surgical literature. The intent of the originator of this review text, M.D. Ram, to provide a comprehensive review of surgery, has been preserved.

Question formats are those used by the United States Medical Licensing Examination (USMLE). The text is organized into fourteen sections. The first thirteen sections deal with specific surgical specialties and statistical evaluation of surgical literature. They contain a variety of question formats. The final section contains only patient management problems and is based upon information presented in preceding sections.

Answers and Comments, explaining the correct answer choice, appears at the end of each section. Answers are referenced, by page number, to major surgical learning resources listed on page xv.

Michael H. Metzler

Acknowledgment

The authors would like to thank Diane McAlpin, BA, for assuring the accuracy of the reference citations.

References

1. Sabiston DC Jr. (ed), *Davis–Christopher Textbook of Surgery,* 14th ed., Philadelphia, WB Saunders Co., 1991.
2. Schwartz SI (ed), *Principles of Surgery,* 6th ed., New York, McGraw-Hill Book Co., 1993.
3. Sabiston DC Jr. (ed), *Sabiston's Essentials of Surgery,* Philadelphia, WB Saunders Co., 1987.
4. Lawrence PF (ed), *Essentials of Surgery,* Baltimore, Williams & Wilkins, 1988.
5. Lawrence PF (ed), *Essentials of Surgical Specialties,* Baltimore, Williams & Wilkins, 1993.
6. Way LW (ed), *Current Surgical Diagnosis & Treatment,* Norwalk, CT, Appleton & Lange, 1994.
7. Wilmore DW, et al. (ed), *Care of the Surgical Patient,* New York, Scientific American, Inc., 1994.
8. American College of Surgeons Committee on Trauma, *Advanced Trauma Life Support,* Chicago, American College of Surgeons, 1993.
9. Dawson-Saunders B, Trapp RG (eds), *Basic and Clinical Biostatistics,* Norwalk, CT, Appleton & Lange, 1990.
10. Pocock SJ (ed), *Clinical Trials: A Practical Approach,* Chichester, England, John Wiley & Sons, 1983.
11. Cook DJ, Jaeschke R, Guyatt GH, et al., Critical Approach of Therapeutic Interventions in the Intensive Care Unit; Human Monoclonal Antibody Treatment in Sepsis, *J. Intensive Care Med* 1992;7:275–282.

A USMLE STEP 2 REVIEW

Surgery

*11*th *Edition*

Basic Surgical Science
Michael H. Metzler

DIRECTIONS (Questions 1 through 5): The group of questions below refers to an accompanying figure with lettered components. For each question, select the ONE lettered component or set of lettered components that is most closely associated with it.

Questions 1 through 4

Figure 1.1 is a pressure recording from the tip of a Swan–Ganz pulmonary artery catheter during its insertion from a right subclavian vein access site to the pulmonary artery. Match the section of the tracing indicated by the letters (A–D) to the description of the tracing.

1. Pulmonary artery (nonwedge position)

2. Right ventricle

3. Subclavian vein or right atrium

4. Pulmonary artery (wedge position)

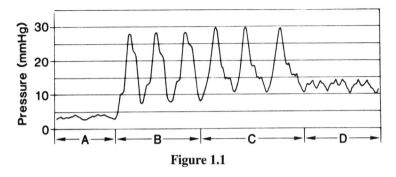

Figure 1.1

Question 5

5. Blood is sampled from the tip of the catheter at each position (Figure 1.1, A–D) and analyzed for oxygen concentration. If this patient has a ventricular–septal defect with left-to-right shunting of blood, a "step-up" in oxygen concentration should be noted between which two cardiac chambers?
   A. A and B
   B. B and C
   C. C and D
   D. B and D
   E. none of the above

DIRECTIONS (Questions 6 through 13): Each of the questions or incomplete statements below is followed by five suggested answers or completions. Select the ONE that is best in each case.

Questions 6 through 8

6. The chest x-ray shown in Figure 1.2 concerns a patient with new frequent runs of ventricular premature contractions (VPCs) and supraventricular tachycardia (SVT). The treatment of choice is
   A. cardioversion
   B. pronestyl
   C. bretylium
   D. verapamil
   E. withdrawal of the catheter loop

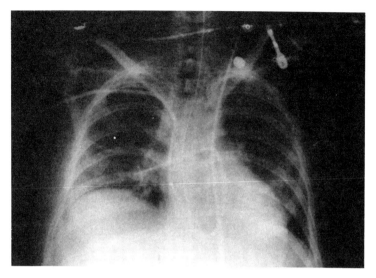

Figure 1.2

7. Ten minutes after the beginning of a blood transfusion, the patient complains of severe chest pain and anxiety. He is found to be hypotensive and tachycardic and to have dark red urine strongly positive for hemoglobin and negative for myoglobin. The patient is MOST likely experiencing
   A. a minor transfusion reaction
   B. a hemolytic transfusion reaction due to bacterial contamination of the unit of blood
   C. a major hemolytic transfusion reaction due to a clerical error in crossmatching this patient or administering blood crossmatched for another patient
   D. a reaction due to platelet antibodies
   E. a myocardial infarction

8. Adequate urine output for adult postoperative surgical patients is greater than
   A. 35 mL/hr regardless of body size
   B. 50 mL/hr regardless of body size
   C. 0.5 mL/kg/hr
   D. 1.0 mL/kg/hr
   E. 1.5 mL/kg/hr

Questions 9 through 13

A 32-year-old female is operated upon to repair an inguinal hernia. During the operation, the skin edges are noted to bleed excessively despite usual hemostasis measures. Postoperatively, the patient developed a wound hematoma and a superficial wound infection.

9. A preoperative history which may suggest a bleeding diathesis includes all of the following EXCEPT
   A. recent, voluntary, dietary weight loss including vitamin supplementation
   B. family history of bleeding post surgery
   C. use of nonsteroidal anti-inflammatory agents (NSAIDs)
   D. bleeding following dental procedures
   E. excessive menstrual flow

10. Coagulation tests in the recovery room showed the following results:

    PT = 12.0 sec   (normal 11.9–12.5 sec)
    APTT = 33.5 sec   (normal 27–35 sec)
    Platelet count = 190,000   (normal 150,000–350,000)

    From this you may conclude
    A. the cause of bleeding must be mechanical (poor technique)
    B. any further hemostatic tests would be a waste of money
    C. a bleeding time might be abnormal
    D. vitamin K therapy is indicated
    E. factor IX replacement is indicated

11. A bleeding time is performed and found to be markedly prolonged. Past bleeding history is not remarkable; the patient underwent an uncomplicated breast reduction procedure 5 years earlier. She now recalls taking a nonprescription sinus medication for the 10 days prior to surgery. A diagnosis which would be supported by the above data is
    A. hemophilia A
    B. hemophilia B
    C. a lupus inhibitor
    D. NSAID medication ingestion
    E. disseminated intravascular coagulation

12. Treatment for this problem may include
   A. vitamin K
   B. platelet transfusion
   C. fresh frozen plasma
   D. cryoprecipitate
   E. search for source of sepsis

13. A patient has had a total gastrectomy for cancer five years previously. She is now found to be anemic with large polymorphonuclear leukocytes on blood smear. A complete work-up fails to find evidence of recurrent tumor. Her condition may be treated with
   A. oral calcium
   B. parenteral calcium
   C. folate only
   D. vitamin B_{12}
   E. cytotoxic chemotherapy

DIRECTIONS (Questions 14 through 26): Each group of questions below consists of lettered headings followed by a list of numbered words, phrases, or statements. For each numbered word, phrase, or statement, select the ONE lettered heading that is most closely associated with it. Each lettered heading may be used once, more than once, or not at all.

Questions 14 through 21

   A. bleeding time
   B. prothombin time (PT)
   C. partial thromboplastin time (PTT)
   D. platelet count
   E. fibrin degradation product (FDP) assay

14. Measures the integrity of the extrinsic coagulation system and common pathway

15. Measures the integrity of the intrinsic coagulation system and common pathway

16. May be normal in patients taking aspirin

17. Measures functional capacity of platelets; it assumes a normal platelet count and other clotting parameters

18. Indicates presence and extent of fibrinolytic activity

19. Used to monitor coumadin therapy

20. Used to monitor heparin therapy

21. Abnormal in cases of vitamin K deficiency

Questions 22 through 26

    A. early septic shock (hypermetabolism)
    B. hypovolemic shock
    C. cardiogenic shock
    D. late septic shock (premorbid)
    E. distributive (neurogenic) shock

22. History of open femur fracture and splenic laceration; blood pressure, 80/70; pulse, 145; skin cool and clammy

23. History of crushing substernal chest pain in 64-year-old man occurring after dinner; blood pressure, 80/70; pulse, 145; skin cool and clammy

24. History of stab wound to the left chest with distended neck veins; cyanosis; blood pressure, 60 by palpation; pulse, 150; skin cool and clammy

25. History of patient falling off a step ladder and sustaining C5 fracture with quadriplegia; blood pressure, 80/40; pulse, 60; skin warm and dry

26. History of hospitalization for fever and urinary tract infection; blood pressure, 80/60; pulse, 100; skin warm and dry

DIRECTIONS (Questions 27 through 30): Each of the questions or incomplete statements below is followed by five suggested answers or completions. Select the ONE that is best in each case.

27. The following statements made regarding anticoagulation therapy of deep venous thrombosis (DVT) in postoperative patients are all true EXCEPT
   A. pneumatic compression stockings are an effective mode of DVT prophylaxis
   B. heparin is an effective mode of DVT prophylaxis
   C. aspirin is a superior agent for DVT prophylaxis
   D. surgery and immobility contribute to development of DVT
   E. patients with antithrombin III (AT III) deficiency are prone to thromboses

28. The following statements made regarding thrombolytic therapy of DVT in postoperative patients are all true EXCEPT
   A. urokinase is effective in treatment of DVT discovered in a patient 3 days postoperatively
   B. urokinase is not used in DVT prophylaxis
   C. urokinase activates plasminogen directly
   D. overdosage may cause hemorrhage
   E. initial treatment is usually followed by heparin

29. The metabolic effects surrounding starvation are characterized by all of the following EXCEPT
   A. mobilization of fat stores, ketosis, and preferential use of ketone bodies for metabolic substrate
   B. exhaustion of carbohydrate stores to use for metabolic substrates
   C. protein is catabolized as substrate for gluconeogenesis for an extended period
   D. decrease in basal metabolic rate
   E. metabolic rate normalized by appropriate feeding

30. The metabolic effects surrounding hypermetabolic state of trauma or sepsis are characterized by all of the following statements EXCEPT

    A. prolonged utilization of fat and protein as metabolic substrate

    B. exhaustion of carbohydrate stores to use for metabolic substrates

    C. protein is catabolized as substrate for gluconeogenesis for an extended period

    D. increase in basal metabolic rate

    E. metabolic rate normalized by appropriate feeding

DIRECTIONS (Questions 31 through 40): Each group of questions below consists of lettered headings followed by a list of numbered words, phrases, or statements. For each numbered word, phrase, or statement, select the ONE lettered heading that is most closely associated with it. Each lettered heading may be used once, more than once, or not at all.

Questions 31 through 40

Match the following hemodynamic measurements and calculations with the choices below.

    A. DO_2 (oxygen delivered to tissues via attachment to hemoglobin)

    B. SvO_2 (oxygen saturation of blood in pulmonary artery)

    C. PaWp (pulmonary artery wedge pressure)

    D. CO (cardiac output)

    E. SaO_2 (oxygen saturation of hemoglobin in arterial blood)

31. Percent of oxygenated hemoglobin in arterial blood

32. Cardiac output/body surface area = cardiac index (CI)

33. Approximated by a pulse oximeter

34. Cardiac output $\times$ (1.38 mL O_2 $\times$ hemoglobin g $\times$ SaO_2) $\times$ 10

35. Mixed venous oxygen saturation

36. Estimate of left ventricular filling pressure

37. Elevated in congestive heart failure (CHF)

38. Not reliable when measured by a pulse oximeter in cases of inhalation burn

39. Low in cardiogenic shock and responsible for this type of shock

40. Difficult to obtain and does not accurately reflect left ventricular filling pressure in cases of mitral valve regurgitation (MVR)

DIRECTIONS (Questions 41 and 42): Each of the questions or incomplete statements below is followed by five suggested answers or completions. Select the ONE that is best in each case.

---

41. Figure 1.3 is a picture of a morbidly obese patient. True statements concerning this disorder include all of the following EXCEPT
   A. "morbidly obese" is defined as 100 pounds greater than ideal body weight
   B. diet therapy is frequently not successful
   C. these patients have a high incidence of respiratory problems following abdominal operations
   D. actual body weight should be used to calculate caloric needs for nutritional support
   E. degenerative joint disease is frequently found

42. A 45-year-old man recovering from penetrating abdominal trauma develops multiple bruises. He has received 14 days of broad spectrum antibiotics and has been on total parenteral nutrition (TPN) for 3 weeks. He appears well otherwise. His prothrombin time (PT) is 19 seconds (normal <13 sec). Hemoglobin and platelet count are normal. A likely reason for his easy bruising and bleeding from venepuncture sites is
   A. disseminated intravascular coagulation
   B. sepsis
   C. vitamin K deficiency
   D. calcium deficiency
   E. magnesium deficiency

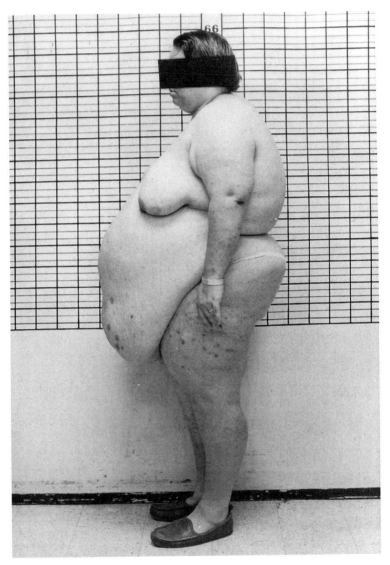

Figure 1.3

DIRECTIONS (Questions 43 through 55): Each group of questions below consists of lettered headings followed by a list of numbered words, phrases, or statements. For each numbered word, phrase, or statement, select the ONE lettered heading that is most closely associated with it. Each lettered heading may be used once, more than once, or not at all.

Questions 43 through 46

Match treatment options with each clinical problem.
  A. Surgical drainage alone, but may also require antibiotics for immunocompromised patients and those with damaged or prosthetic heart valves
  B. systemic antibiotic therapy without surgery
  C. hyperbaric oxygen
  D. topical antibiotics

43. Treatment for 3-cm cutaneous abscess

44. Treatment for cellulitis with lymphangitis, fever, and prostration.

45. Treatment for nosocomial pneumonia

46. Treatment for thrombosed hemorrhoid

Questions 47 through 51

  A. approximately 10%
  B. less than 10%
  C. approximately 50%
  D. greater than 75%
  E. unknown

47. The chances that patients with classical complaints of cholelithiasis and findings of gallstones on ultrasound will have relief of their complaints by cholecystectomy

48. The chances that an average risk woman will develop breast cancer

49. The chances for 5-year survival following surgical removal of pancreatic cancer of the body of the gland

50. Expected survival for a young child with favorable stage and grade of Wilms' tumor treated by multimodality therapy

51. Percentage of pancreatitis associated with either alcohol abuse or cholelithiasis

Questions 52 through 55

Proper tetanus treatment includes which of the following choices in each clinical situation?
- **A.** tetanus immune globulin (TIG)
- **B.** tetanus toxoid usually given as DT (diphtheria toxoid + tetanus)
- **C.** no additional tetanus therapy indicated
- **D.** TIG + DT, followed by complete immunization

52. An elderly immigrant migrant worker who develops tetanus following a neglected puncture wound

53. Given every ten years as a "booster"

54. A laboratory technician cut her hand on a clean glass slide; last tetanus immunization 4 years ago; full prior immunization

55. A farmer sustained a puncture wound in his barnyard; last tetanus immunization 4 years ago; full prior immunization

---

DIRECTIONS (Questions 56 through 59): Each of the questions or incomplete statements below is followed by five suggested answers or completions. Select the ONE that is best in each case.

Questions 56 and 57

56. The statements below regarding bowel obstruction are all true EXCEPT
  A. abdominal distention usually noted on physical exam and dilated loops of bowel usually present on abdominal x-ray
  B. likely to require operation if not promptly resolved
  C. treated by bowel stimulants (eg, neostigmine)
  D. characterized by high-pitched, tinkling bowel sounds
  E. characterized by intermittent spasms of pain interspersed with relatively pain-free periods

57. The statements below regarding ileus are all true EXCEPT
  A. abdominal distention usually noted on physical exam and loops of bowel with gas throughout the GI tract present on abdominal x-ray
  B. usually responds to supportive measures and correction of underlying disorders
  C. treated by bowel stimulants (eg, neostigmine)
  D. characterized by hypoactive bowel sounds
  E. not characterized by intermittent spasms of pain interspersed with relatively pain-free periods

Questions 58 and 59

58. Compared to the patient at point "B," the patient who is shown at point "A" in Figure 1.4 is best described as
  A. hyperdynamic
  B. volume depleted
  C. normal
  D. abnormal cardiac function
  E. bradycardic

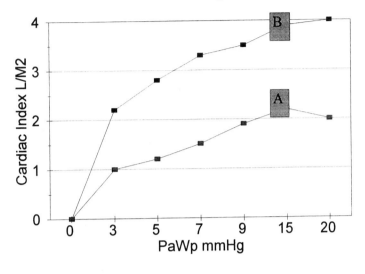

Figure 1.4

59. Therapy that may change cardiac performance from point "A" toward "B" include all of the following EXCEPT
    A. dopamine infusion
    B. Lasix 40 mg
    C. dobutamine
    D. digoxin therapy
    E. warm patient if hypothermic

Basic Surgical Science

Answers and Comments

1. (C)

2. (B)

3. (A)

4. **(D)** Answers 1 through 4 refer to portions of a pressure tracing from the tip of a pulmonary artery catheter encountered during routine, uncomplicated placement. Respiratory artifact has been minimized. Part A shows a pressure tracing of the intrathoracic venous system proximal to the right ventricle. Part B shows the characteristic change to the systolic and diastolic fluctuations of pressure within the right ventricle. Part C indicates that the catheter has moved into the pulmonary outflow tract. Note the rise in diastolic baseline between "B" and "C." Part D indicates the characteristic waveform of pulmonary artery wedge (occlusion) pressure. (**Ref. 7,** Part II, Sect. 1, pp. 7–19)

5. **(A)** A ventricular–septal defect (VSD) with left-to-right shunting of blood would cause an unexpected oxygen content increase in right ventricle blood. Without such a shunt, there is no increase in blood oxygen concentration between the right atrium and right ventricle. If blood is aspirated from a catheter wedged in the pulmonary artery, oxygenated blood from the left atrium may be drawn back into the sample producing a step up in oxygen content. This step up is not due to a VSD. (**Ref. 7,** Part II, Sect. 2, p. 4)

6. **(E)** There is a loop in the pulmonary artery catheter as it passes through the right atrium and ventricle. The removal of this stimulus is the correct treatment. (**Ref. 7,** Part II, Sect. 1, pp. 11–12)

7. **(C)** Major hemolytic transfusion reactions usually begin shortly after the start of administration of the blood (as little as 20 mL of transfusion). Hematuria, hypotension, and chest and muscle aches are often present. Disseminated intravascular coagulation (DIC) may also result. The usual cause of a major hemolytic transfusion reaction is clerical—wrong specimen collected, blood administered to the wrong patient, etc. Minor transfusion reactions (fever, urticaria) are usually due to leukocytes present in the unit and platelet antibodies. They do not produce hemolysis. It is rare that blood is contaminated by bacteria if collected, stored, and administered correctly. (**Ref. 1,** pp. 96–97; **Ref. 6,** pp. 56–57)

8. **(C)** Under routine conditions, adequate urine output for adults is greater than 0.5 mL/kg/hr. There are occasions where a greater output may be desired (such as patients with myoglobin in their urine). Elderly patients who have been chronically taking diuretics may not attain adequate urine output without diuretic therapy. (**Ref. 1,** pp. 69–70; **Ref. 7,** Part II, Sect. 6, p. 3)

9. **(A)** Family history of bleeding as well as excessive menstrual flow or bleeding problems following dental work are good indicators of hereditary bleeding disorders. Use of NSAIDs suggest the possibility of an acquired bleeding disorder. Diet restriction with vitamin supplementation does not suggest an etiology of bleeding. (**Ref. 1,** pp. 101–104)

10. **(C)** PT and PTT are normal. This does not suggest a soluble coagulation factor deficiency or presence of an inhibitor as the cause of bleeding. Factor IX replacement is not indicated. Platelet number is normal, but platelet function was not measured and may be the problem. (**Ref. 1,** pp. 104–105)

11. **(D)**   It is likely that the sinus medication contained aspirin or some other NSAID. This would be most consistent with the history of a competent and tested coagulation system in the past and a recently acquired coagulopathy. (**Ref. 1,** p. 501)

12. **(B)**   Depending upon the bleeding severity, platelet transfusion may be indicated. All other therapies suggested would not improve the platelet dysfunction. Platelets are manufactured and released at a continuous rate. Different NSAIDs act at different points in the platelet and remain effective for varying time periods. (**Ref. 1,** p. 501)

13. **(D)**   The patient is most likely suffering from megaloblastic anemia caused by B_{12} malabsorption due to absence of intrinsic factor (IF). IF is made by the gastric mucosa. Vitamin B_{12} is usually given parenterally to obviate the need for intrinsic factor. Folate should not be given until B_{12} is present or metabolic nerve damage may ensue. (**Ref. 6,** p. 474)

14. **(B)**   The PT primarily measures function of components of the extrinsic pathway. (**Ref. 1,** p. 104)

15. **(C)**   The PTT primarily measures components of the intrinsic pathway. The intrinsic and extrinsic pathways function together in vivo. Their separation is mostly a laboratory phenomena, but valuable for monitoring anticoagulant therapy and understanding coagulopathies. (**Ref. 1,** p. 104)

16. **(D)**   Although the platelet count may be normal, platelet function may be affected by aspirin. Bleeding time is an assessment of platelet function. (**Ref. 1,** p. 104)

17. **(A)**   In order for a bleeding time to be accurate, the platelet count must be ≥ 100,000. (**Ref. 1,** pp. 103–104)

18. **(E)**   Fibrin degradation products circulating in the plasma indicate clot dissolution due to fibrinolytic activity. (**Ref. 1,** p. 104)

19. **(B)**   The PT is used to monitor the vitamin K-dependent clotting factors II, VII, IX, and X. The half-life of factor VII is much shorter than factors II, IX, or X, making it the limiting factor al-

tering the extrinsic before the intrinsic coagulation system. (**Ref. 1,** p. 104)

20. **(C)**   The PTT is used to monitor heparin therapy. (**Ref. 1,** p. 102)

21. **(B)**   See answer 19. (**Ref. 1,** p. 104)

22. **(B)**   The patient is hypotensive, tachycardic, and has skin signs of decreased perfusion. With the history of significant trauma, there is sufficient information to make a diagnosis of hypovolemic shock. (**Ref. 6,** p. 187)

23. **(C)**   The history and physical findings are classical for cardiogenic shock. (**Ref. 6,** pp. 190–191)

24. **(C)**   Cardiogenic shock related to pericardial tamponade is described in this example. This is sometimes called cardiac compressive shock. (**Ref. 6,** p. 189)

25. **(E)**   Neurogenic shock secondary to acute spinal cord injury with loss of sympathetic tone is described. (**Ref. 6,** p. 192)

26. **(A)**   The hyperdynamic state with warm extremities and elevated cardiac output is characteristic of this type of shock. The most recent terminology refers to these findings as systemic inflammatory response syndrome (SIRS) in patients whose septic hypotension is reversed by volume infusion alone. The term "septic shock" is reserved for situations which require inotropic or vasopressor support. (**Ref. 6,** pp. 192–193)

27. **(C)**   While some studies show aspirin to be superior to no treatment in regard to DVT prophylaxis following hip replacement surgery, aspirin is not generally thought to be as good a venous prophylactic agent as others available. Aspirin's antiplatelet actions appear to be much more effective in preventing arterial than venous thrombosis. Pneumatic compression hose, leg elevation, and ambulation are means of increasing venous flow and decreasing stasis. Heparin acts through amplification of the naturally occurring antithrombin factor AT III. The so-called "mini-dose" regimen acts by inhibiting activated factor X—the common pathway for intrinsic and extrinsic coagulation systems. Virchow's

triad of stasis, hypercoagulability, and venous endothelial damage form the basis for DVT risk factors. Surgery and immobility are two specific risk factors. Antithrombin III (AT III) is a naturally occurring clotting inhibitor. Its activity is greatly enhanced by heparin. (**Ref. 1,** p. 102; **Ref. 6,** pp. 792, 788, 793)

28. **(A)** Urokinase activates plasminogen directly and is effective in the treatment of early DVT. It is usually contraindicated in the patient who is recently postoperative for fear or lysis of normal clot at the operative site. Urokinase is NOT approved for DVT prophylaxis. Initial fibrinolytic therapy is usually followed by heparin anticoagulation. Overdosage may cause hemorrhage. (**Ref. 6,** pp. 793, 795; **Ref. 7,** Part VII, Sect. 1, p. 10; **Ref. 7,** Part VII, Sect. 8, p. 18)

29. **(C)** After the first few days of starvation, the body adapts to economic utilization of fat stores. Carbohydrate stores, in the form of starches, are exhausted early. Starvation is accompanied by lethargy and a decrease in metabolic rate. Feeding completely reverses the metabolic alterations of starvation. Such is not the case with sepsis. (**Ref. 6,** pp. 149–150)

30. **(E)** Sepsis produces a hyperdynamic state. Carbohydrate stores are exhausted early, as in starvation. However, protein is used for gluconeogenesis far beyond the initial few days. This hypermetabolic response is mediated by a host of biologically active molecules, and the state may continue for weeks. Unlike starvation, feeding does not reverse the process. (**Ref. 6,** pp. 152–153)

31. **(E)** The SaO_2 is the percentage of oxygenated hemoglobin present, as compared with measured normal hemoglobin. (**Ref. 7,** Part II, Sect. 1, p. 4)

32. **(D)** Cardiac output divided by body surface area (BSA) = CI. Indexing is an attempt to better relate hemodynamic parameters to body size rather than absolute values regardless of size. Cardiac output is usually measured by thermodilution technique. (**Ref. 7,** Part II, Sect. 1, pp. 16–18)

33. (E) Pulse oximeters do not take into account dyshemoglobins and therefore approximate the SaO_2. A co-oximeter (laboratory instrument used in blood gas analysis) measures other hemoglobins present and provides a more accurate SaO_2 measurement. (**Ref. 8,** p. 249)

34. (A) Oxygen delivered to the tissues (DO_2) is a function of oxygen content of the blood and cardiac output. Only the portion of oxygen attached to hemoglobin is accounted for in the equation given. There is also oxygen dissolved in the plasma, but this is insignificant in patients inspiring normal oxygen concentrations. (**Ref. 7,** Part II, Sect. 2, p. 4)

35. (B) Mixed venous oxygen saturation is obtained by measurement of pulmonary artery blood. Blood from this area is a "mixed" return from the superior and inferior vena cavae, as well as from the coronary sinus of the heart. (**Ref. 7,** Part II, Sect. 1, pp. 18–19)

36. (C) The pulmonary capillary wedge pressure is obtained by temporarily occluding the proximal branch of a pulmonary artery and measuring the pressure in the capillary bed of the lung distal to that occlusion. That pressure is related to the filling pressure of the left atrium, as well as the left ventricle. (**Ref. 7,** Part II, Sect. 1, pp. 16–17)

37. (C) In cases of CHF, the heart is unable to handle the venous return. The wedge pressure is elevated reflecting this. (**Ref. 7,** Part II, Sect. 1, pp. 16–17)

38. (E) Abnormal hemoglobins (such as carboxyhemoglobin and methemoglobin) are usually not measured by pulse oximetry. Carbon monoxide poisoning (as with inhalation burns) may give spuriously high SaO_2 readings due to elevated level of dyshemoglobins. (**Ref. 8,** p. 249)

39. (D) Although values of other parameters may be low in the case of cardiogenic shock, they are a reflection of the primary underlying problem—low cardiac output. A low cardiac output or index defines this disorder. (**Ref. 7,** Part I, Sect. 1, pp. 9–14)

40. (C) In cases of MVR, there is conduction of left ventricular systolic pressure retrograde into the pulmonary artery because of the incompetent valve making PaWp difficult to measure and interpret. (**Ref. 7,** Part II, Sect. 1, p. 13)

41. (D) Ideal body weight based on calculations or nomograms incorporating height should be used for estimating resting energy expenditure (REE). Estimates of REE based upon actual body weight will result in overfeeding. (**Ref. 7,** Part I, Sect. 12, p. 8)

42. (C) Antibiotics are likely to suppress normal gut flora that produce vitamin K. Most TPN preparations do not include vitamin K. These two factors frequently lead to coagulation defects manifest by easy bruising and prolonged PT. The other choices are unlikely or do not primarily affect coagulation. (**Ref. 1,** pp. 89–90)

43. (A) Surgical drainage is the preferred treatment. In most cases, antibiotic therapy is not indicated. (**Ref. 6,** p. 106)

44. (B) Intravenous antibiotic therapy is indicated here. There is usually no need for surgery unless an abscess forms. The intravenous route is chosen because of the severity of the response to infection. (**Ref. 6,** p. 96)

45. (B) Intravenous antibiotic therapy is also indicated here. Surgical therapy is reserved for complications of abscess, empyema, or bronchiectasis. (**Ref. 7,** Part II, Sect. 7, p. 2)

46. (A) Enucleation of the clot from an acutely thrombosed hemorrhoid is frequently curative. Antibiotics are usually not used even as adjunctive therapy. (**Ref. 1,** p. 963)

47. (D) Removal of the gallbladder either by laparoscopic or by open technique is curative in over 90% of patients who present with classical symptoms of gallbladder pain and have stones. (**Ref. 6,** p. 548)

48. (A) Approximately 1 in 8 to 10 women will develop breast cancer. Women with maternal premenopausal breast cancer history or biopsy-proven hyperplasia have a significantly higher risk. (**Ref. 6,** pp. 294–295)

49. (B) Pancreatic resection for cancer of the ampulla of the bile duct may result in 5-year survival rates of 35%, but similar survivors for cancer that arises in the body of the gland are about 5%. The hospital mortality of a Whipple procedure has decreased in recent years; death is usually due to recurrent disease. (**Ref. 6,** p. 588)

50. (D) Current survival for multimodality therapy (surgery plus chemotherapy and/or radiation therapy) of nephroblastoma exceeds 85%. This is a marked improvement over surgery alone. (**Ref. 6,** p. 1237)

51. (D) Approximately 80% of pancreatitis is associated with either cholelithiasis or alcohol use. Many other causes collectively comprise the remaining 20%. (**Ref. 6,** p. 569)

52. (D) TIG is indicated to ameliorate the present case of tetanus. DT begins the immunization protocol. It is likely that this patient never received full immunization or his immune system has no amnestic immune response. Having a full-blown case of tetanus does NOT confer immunity. (**Ref. 1,** p. 290)

53. (B) DT is routinely given every ten years to maintain immune status. (**Ref. 1,** p. 290)

54. (C) The injury represents a clean wound; immunization is current. This wound is low-risk for tetanus complications. No specific immune therapy is indicated. (**Ref. 1,** p. 290)

55. (B) The injury represents a tetanus-prone wound; immunization is current. This is a high-risk wound for tetanus complications. If the last DT booster had been given within the last year, no further immune treatment would be necessary. The combination of high-risk wound and 4 years since last DT make DT immunization recommended. The history of full prior immunization negates need for passive immune therapy (TIG). (**Ref. 1,** p. 290)

56. (C) Bowel stimulants are contraindicated in obstruction and usually of no use in cases of ileus. Distention and dilated loops of bowel are common to both ileus and bowel obstruction. Bowel obstruction is treated by operation if it does not resolve spontaneously; ileus is not usually treated operatively. Tinkling bowel sounds are characteristic of early bowel obstruction prior to the onset of ischemia. Rushes may also be heard and coincide with crampy pain. As ischemia and infarction progress, bowel sounds decrease. Periods of pain interspersed with relatively pain-free times is the definition of colic and characteristic of obstruction. (**Ref. 6,** pp. 442, 446, 448, 617; **Ref. 7,** Part II, Sect. 9, pp. 5–6)

57. **(C)** Ileus is usually a reflection of the postoperative state or a metabolic abnormality. Correction of the underlying cause will result in its resolution. Bowel stimulants are usually of no use in cases of ileus. (**Ref. 7,** Part II, Sect. 9, pp. 4–5)

58. **(D)** The lower cardiac function curve shows abnormal, hypodynamic cardiac function in comparison to the upper curve. There is adequate filling pressure as witnessed by a PaWp of 15 mm Hg. (**Ref. 7,** Part I, Sect. 4, p. 11)

59. **(B)** Use of an inotrope (digoxin, dobutamine, or dopamine) shifts the hypodynamic cardiac function curve toward the upper, more normal curve. Heat, in the case of hypothermia, will add inotropic stimulus and vasodilation—both shift the dysfunctional curve upward. Use of a diuretic will simply change the PaWp and CI to lower values on the same function curve. (**Ref. 7,** Part II, Sect. 2, pp. 5–7)

2

Statistics and Clinical Literature Interpretation
Jeffrey O. Phillips

DIRECTIONS (Questions 1 through 19): Each of the questions or incomplete statements below is followed by five suggested answers or completions. Select the ONE that is best in each case.

Note that questions contain fictitious drug names.

1. When preparing a trial that will evaluate two surgical techniques (eg, inguinal hernia repair technique A, "the standard technique," and inguinal hernia repair technique B), which of the following statements would be the appropriate way to state the nondirectional alternative hypothesis?
   A. surgical technique A is better than surgical technique B
   B. surgical technique B is not better than surgical technique A
   C. there is a difference between surgical technique A and surgical technique B
   D. surgical technique B is not different from surgical technique A
   E. surgical technique A is not different from surgical technique B

2. Which of the following is not an appropriate definition of hypothesis?
  A. a preconceived idea
  B. a proven explanation for a group of phenomena
  C. the basis for reasoning and experimentation
  D. an assumption
  E. a supposition used to explain something

3. A "controlled" trial is so named because
  A. the experimenter is overseeing the assignment of subjects
  B. the experimenter has included a therapy or procedure with a known or expected outcome to compare to the experimental therapy or procedure
  C. the study is designed in a prospective fashion to permit full oversight over the collection of data
  D. the experimenter is minimizing bias by including a randomization sequence for the assignment of patients to the different study arms
  E. the bias of the experimenter is kept from influencing patient selection through blinding

4. You are reviewing a study which compared lincocillin with maximicin in the treatment of nosocomial pneumonia. Lincocillin is the standard therapy, and maximicin is a newer treatment. The study was a randomized clinical trial which enrolled 104 subjects (50 in the lincocillin arm, 54 in the maximicin arm). The clinical cure rate was 78% for lincocillin and 86% for maximicin, $p = 0.12$. Assuming that the study was performed appropriately, what can be concluded?
  A. the study has failed to demonstrate a statistically significant difference in clinical cure rate between lincocillin and maximicin
  B. there was a trend toward improved clinical cure rates with maximicin
  C. there is an 88% likelihood that the failure to detect a statistically significant difference between lincocillin and maximicin was due to chance alone
  D. there is an 88% likelihood that the failure to detect a statistically significant difference between lincocillin and maximicin was due to the relatively low sample size
  E. a larger sample size would have led to a smaller type I error

5. Which of the following appropriately describes type I error?
   A. it is the error made when you have statistically concluded that a difference does exist when in reality a difference does not exist
   B. it is the error of not finding a difference when one really does exist
   C. type I error is also referred to as beta error
   D. 1 − power = type I error
   E. power − type II error = type I error

6. When trying to determine whether a study is scientifically acceptable, one is asking about the study's
   A. internal validity
   B. power
   C. alpha error
   D. statistical analysis
   E. alpha and beta error

7. In order to determine the statistically appropriate sample size for a study, it is important to know the acceptable type I and type II error rates and the related f value, the percentage of success expected on the standard treatment, and
   A. the desirable power
   B. whether there will be more than two treatments in different groups
   C. the percent of success expected on the experimental treatment
   D. the expected standard deviations of the study population with regard to the dependent variable being evaluated
   E. whether there will be two treatments in different groups

8. You are reviewing a randomized clinical trial of the fictitious drugs emfatuon vs. trosopidol in the reduction of postoperative ileus. Emfatuon was statistically better at reducing ileus than trosopidol (p = 0.02). You plan to use emfatuon to minimize postoperative ileus in one of your own patients. Which of the following information will give you the treatment effect you could expect in your patient?
   A. the mean effect, gathered from those patients who responded to emfatuon with a significant reduction in ileus
   B. 95% confidence intervals built around the mean effect emfatuon had on ileus

C. there is a 98% chance that emfatuon will work in your patient $(1 - 0.02 = 0.98)$

D. the expected effect of emfatuon on postoperative ileus can be determined by using power

E. the mean ± standard error of the mean

9. A study is designed to compare the total cost of care associated with a group of patients who receive resuscitation to "Shoemaker's criteria" and a group who does not. The accepted type I error is 5%; type II error is 20%. A sample size calculation indicates that 180 patients per arm are required to detect a 15% reduction in the cost of care for the "Shoemaker group." The study is performed, and an interim statistical evaluation at 110 patients per arm fails to detect a difference in the cost of care between the groups. The following interim data are made available:

Total cost of care–Shoemaker group $122,000
Total cost of care–other group $136,000   p = 0.113

What can be concluded at this time about this study?

A. the interim evaluation showed little likelihood of a difference being detected at study completion

B. since the power of the study is 80%, there is still a 20% chance that a statistically significant difference will be detected

C. if the study were terminated at the interim evaluation, the type II error would exceed 20%

D. if the study were terminated at the interim evaluation, the type I error would remain at 5%

E. since the p value of the statistic is 0.11, there is still an 11% chance that a statistically significant difference will be detected

10. A prospective, randomized, controlled clinical trial is designed to compare gentamicin/clindamycin to newercillin in the treatment of sepsis of abdominal origin. Newercillin has activity against most anaerobes and aerobic bacteria, including *Pseudomonas aeruginosa*. Newercillin is to be given at the recommended dosage for serious infections 2 g q8h and gentamicin 80 mg q8h/clindamycin 900 mg q8h. The study is to be double-blinded (the patients who receive newercillin will get a dummy bag to correspond with the clindamycin). Patients who have a >90% predicted risk of mortality and those receiving concomitant antibiotics are excluded from entry. The accepted type I error is 5%; type II error is 20%. A sample size calculation indicates that 120 patients per arm are required to detect a 20% reduction in "significant morbidity" or mortality. Are there any flaws you can detect in this study?

    A. the study size is too large to be feasibly performed
    B. there is no provision to make sure that the groups are comparable at study entry
    C. the experimental and control groups are not appropriate
    D. the type II error is too high
    E. the likelihood of a difference being detected is too low

11. A randomized study is designed to compare pain control in a group of postoperative laparascopic cholecystectomy patients (some of whom will receive zetorolac and some of whom will receive olbuprofen). There will be approximately 50 patients per arm. The patients will evaluate their pain on a pain index which goes from 1 to 10 (1 being no pain and 10 being excruciating pain). What type of data is being obtained?

    A. continuous data
    B. nominal data
    C. ordinal data
    D. interval data
    E. ratio data

12. In the pain study described in question #11, what would be an appropriate statistic to use for determining whether a difference in pain control exists between zetorolac and olbuprofen?

    A. Mann–Whitney U test
    B. paired t-test
    C. unpaired t-test

D. Fisher exact test
E. Wilcoxon signed ranks test

13. A pilot study is performed prior to the clinical trial of zetorolac and olbuprofen (see question #11). There are 18 subjects enrolled (8 in the zetorolac arm and 10 in the olbuprofen arm). What would be an appropriate statistic to use for determining whether a difference in pain control exists between zetorolac and olbuprofen?
A. Mann–Whitney U test
B. paired t-test
C. unpaired t-test
D. Fisher exact test
E. Wilcoxon signed ranks test

14. The alternative hypothesis
A. assumes that the treatment groups are different
B. assumes that the treatment groups are not different
C. is usually directional
D. assumes that the treatment groups are the same
E. is also known as the primary hypothesis

15. A decreased sample size would be required for which of the following?
A. a beta of 0.1 instead of 0.2
B. an alpha 0.05 instead of 0.1
C. a small expected difference between two study treatments
D. a meta-analysis
E. a study that employs a crossover instead of a parallel design

16. A study is designed to measure the oxygen utilization (VO_2) after two different treatment plans (A and B). Plan A is to push oxygen delivery to >600 mL/min/m². Plan B is to maintain the PcWP at >12 mm Hg. One hundred twenty subjects are enrolled in the study (57 on plan A and 63 on plan B). The mean maximal VO_2 achieved for each plan was 148 mL/min/m² (plan A) and 127 mL/min/m² (plan B). An alpha of 0.05 and a beta of 0.2 are set. What type of data is being obtained?

    A. continuous data
    B. nominal data
    C. interval data
    D. ordinal data
    E. discrete data

17. Considering the study outlined in question #16, what would be an appropriate statistical test to use for determining whether a significant difference in VO_2 exists between plan A and plan B?

    A. Mann–Whitney U test
    B. paired t-test
    C. unpaired t-test
    D. Fisher exact test
    E. Wilcoxon signed ranks test

18. The results of appropriate statistical testing (for the study outlined in question #16) reveal the following:

The mean maximal VO_2 achieved for: Plan A was 148 mL/min/m²
    Plan B was 127 mL/min/m²
    $p = 0.035$

What can be concluded?

    A. there is no statistically significant difference between plan A and plan B
    B. there is a small statistically significant difference between plan A and plan B
    C. there is a statistically significant difference between plan A and plan B

D. there is a statistically significant difference between plan A and plan B, but it must be acknowledged that there is a 20% likelihood that this difference was due to chance alone

E. there is no statistically significant difference between plan A and plan B, but there may be a clinically significant difference

19. If a statistically significant difference is found between two therapies, what else is known?

A. the type II error was probably low

B. alpha was set at 0.05 or 0.01

C. the null hypothesis was accepted

D. the alternative hypothesis was accepted

E. the null hypothesis was rejected

Statistics and Clinical Literature Interpretation

Answers and Comments

1. **(C)** Generally, one of two conclusions can be drawn after comparing two (or more) different techniques (or therapies, etc.) in a study. The researcher will either find a difference between the different techniques (or therapies, etc.) or not. The researcher should state the study question in the form of statistical hypotheses. These hypotheses should specifically reflect the two potential conclusions. They are the null hypothesis and the alternative hypothesis. The *null* hypothesis states that there is no difference between the items being compared. The *alternative* hypothesis states that there is a difference between the items being compared. The alternative hypothesis can be directional or nondirectional. A directional alternative hypothesis not only states that there is a difference but also states the expected direction of the difference (ie, repair technique A is better than repair technique B). More frequently, however, no specific direction of difference will be noted (ie, there is a difference between surgical technique A and surgical technique B). In this case, the alternative hypothesis is nondirectional. (**Ref. 9,** p. 93; **Ref. 10,** pp. 198–199)

2. **(B)** Although hypothesis is used informally as a colloquial term (in which case it has a variety of meanings), it has a very specific

and important meaning to those interested in statistics. A theory is a proven explanation for a group of phenomena. (**Ref. 9,** p. 93)

3. **(B)** When a trial is "controlled," the therapy being studied is being compared to a therapy whose effect on an illness is known or well-described. A trial that employs a negative control (frequently called a placebo-controlled trial) uses a control technique with no effect on the illness. A trial that compares the therapy being studied to an active therapy, usually the gold standard, is using a control technique with a positive effect on the illness and thus employs a positive control. (**Ref. 9,** p. 12)

4. **(A)** There is a tendency to read more into the statistical analysis than is intended. If statistical analysis produces a p value greater than that point set prior to the study commencement (usually 0.05), then the study has failed to demonstrate a statistically significant difference between the therapies. (**Ref. 9,** p. 94)

5. **(A)** Type I error is the error of concluding that there is a difference between two (or more) treatments when in reality there is no difference. Conventionally, most are willing to allow a 5% chance of making this type of an error, hence an alpha of 0.05. Type I error is sometimes called alpha error; however, this is a misnomer as there is no such term in statistics as alpha error. (**Ref. 9,** pp. 95–96; **Ref. 10,** pp. 125–129)

6. **(C)** The internal validity pertains to the appropriateness of the study itself. For a study to possess internal validity, such factors as methods, materials, design, and statistical analysis should be found to be acceptable. (**Ref. 11,** pp. 275–282)

7. **(C)** The calculation of appropriate sample size is as important to a study as the enrollment of subjects. However, it is often thought to be too complex to calculate. Nothing could be further from the truth. One need only have four pieces of information; the only one missing is the percentage of success expected in the experimental group. (**Ref. 9,** pp. 118–119; **Ref. 10,** pp. 123–141)

8. **(B)** We are so oriented to averages (means) that we might expect a patient treated with emfatuon to do as well as the mean value in the study. Appropriate assessment of treatment effect in-

volves the use of confidence intervals. Ninety-five percent confidence intervals allow you to create a zone of expectation around the mean in which 95% of patients treated with such a therapy (in this case emfatuon) will fall. (Other size confidence intervals such as 90% or 99% can be set, but 95% is conventional.) (**Ref. 9,** pp. 96–97; **Ref. 10,** pp. 187, 206–210)

9. **(C)** A determination of type II error is based on the number of patients enrolled in a trial. If fewer patients are enrolled than the prespecified quantity and a difference is not detected, the type II error will be higher than that specified in the trial design (in this case higher than 20%). (**Ref. 9,** pp. 95–96; **Ref. 10,** pp. 125–129, 132–133)

10. **(B)** For a study to be considered internally valid, various characteristics about the study itself must be found to be appropriate (see question #6 above). One of these characteristics is that the therapies being studied must be considered comparable (this includes factors such as drug choice and drug dosage regimen). Comparability is determined from prior research (both animal and human) and cannot be completely known prior to the study (or there would be no reason to perform the study). A common breach of comparability involves drug dosage (especially in critically ill patients). Aminoglycosides have been studied extensively and must be dosed to achieve or exceed specific concentrations. This study is designed to provide outdated "standard aminoglycoside" dosages and therefore does not ensure comparability. (**Ref. 11,** pp. 275–282)

11. **(C)** An initial part of determining the appropriate statistical test is to determine the level of data with which you will be working. Nominal data (the lowest level of data) has no inherent rank. Ordinal data has some rank but the rankings are not arithmetically meaningful. Interval (and ratio) data are arithmetically rankable (eg, 2 is twice as much as 1 and half as much as 4, etc.). (**Ref. 9,** pp. 21–23, 38, 50, 56)

12. **(A)** After determining the level of data, choosing an appropriate statistical test can be accomplished by knowing: (1) how many treatments are being compared, (2) in how many groups of subjects, and (3) are the data normally distributed? In this case there

are two treatments being compared in two different groups of subjects, and the data are normally distributed (sample sizes of approximately ≥25 usually yield a normal distribution). An appropriate statistical test for this setting is the Mann–Whitney U test. (**Ref. 9,** pp. 116–118)

13. **(A)**   The only change from #12 above is the lower number of patients that will produce the potential for a distribution of data that is not normal (for the population in question); therefore, a more rigorous test is required. In this case the appropriate statistical test is a Fisher exact test. (**Ref. 9,** pp. 150–151)

14. **(A)**   It is standard to think of one hypothesis in relation to a study. In reality, there are two hypothesis statements that should be constructed as a part of the methodology of any study. They include the null hypothesis and the alternative hypothesis. The alternative hypothesis assumes that there *is* a difference between one of the treatments of a study and the other treatment(s) being studied (see question #1). (**Ref. 9,** p. 93; **Ref. 10,** pp. 198–199)

15. **(E)**   Appropriate sample size is dependent upon several factors (as mentioned in question #7), most of which aim to minimize the bias introduced by intersubject variation. Study design is not often thought of as affecting sample size. However, in a crossover study the number of subjects required is reduced, since each subject serves as his/her own control and as such serves to minimize bias. (**Ref. 9,** p. 13; **Ref. 10,** pp. 110–122)

16. **(A)**   In addition to the arithmetical character of data, it can be classified as discrete or continuous. Continuous data are those that are infinitely divisible, having no specifically defined points. Examples of continuous data are measurements of weight, length, time, etc. (**Ref. 9,** p. 22)

17. (C) The unpaired t-test is the appropriate statistic for evaluating these data. The key factors that determine which statistical test should be employed are:

1. Level of data?	Interval or greater
2. How many treatments are being compared?	Two
3. In how many groups of subjects?	Two different groups
4. Are the data normally distributed?	Yes

(**Ref. 9**, pp. 114–115; **Ref. 10,** pp. 196, 200–202)

18. (C) Since there are two hypothesis statements, there can be only one of two conclusions. There either is or is not a difference between "plan A and plan B." In this case, since the a priori designated statistical point of difference was 0.05 and the result of statistical testing was $p = 0.035$, there is a difference between "plan A and plan B." (**Ref. 9,** p. 93)

19. (E) If a statistically significant difference is not found between two treatments, then there has been a failure to reject the null hypothesis. It should be noted that failing to reject the null hypothesis is not the same as accepting the null hypothesis. In statistical science it is never possible to accept the null hypothesis. (**Ref. 9,** p. 93)

3

Abdominal Surgery
Brent W. Miedema

DIRECTIONS (Questions 1 through 69): Each of the questions or incomplete statements below is followed by five suggested answers or completions. Select the ONE that is best in each case.

Questions 1 through 10

1. The MOST important finding in the diagnosis of appendicitis is
   A. vomiting
   B. fever
   C. leukocytosis
   D. right lower quadrant tenderness
   E. referred rebound tenderness (Rovsing's sign)

2. The abdominal x-ray in Figure 3.1 is consistent with which clinical situation?
   A. intra-abdominal adhesions
   B. annular pancreas
   C. peritonitis
   D. volvulus
   E. intussusception

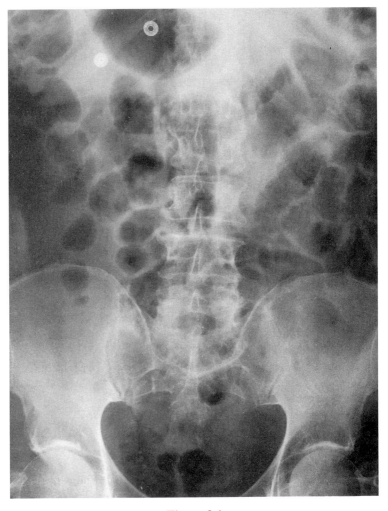

Figure 3.1

3. Splenectomy is commonly indicated in all of the following EX-CEPT
   A. immune thrombocytopenic purpura
   B. hypersplenism associated with cirrhosis
   C. hereditary spherocytosis
   D. grade IV splenic injury and multitrauma
   E. splenic tumor

4. The MOST frequent indication for surgery in Crohn's disease of the small intestine is
   A. internal fistula
   B. intra-abdominal abscess
   C. gastrointestinal bleeding
   D. partial obstruction
   E. abdominal mass

5. The MOST common site of intestinal obstruction due to cholecystoenteric fistula is the
   A. pylorus
   B. duodenum
   C. jejunum
   D. ileum
   E. sigmoid colon

6. The MOST important technical aspect when establishing a permanent ileostomy is
   A. placing the stoma on the right side
   B. fashioning a long segment of ileum that will hang down into the ileostomy bag
   C. placement of a well-fitting ileostomy bag at the time of operation
   D. creating an ileal pouch to act as a reservoir
   E. primary maturation of the ileostomy

7. Which of the following polyps of the colon and rectum is MOST likely to contain a malignancy?
   A. villous adenoma
   B. juvenile polyp
   C. tubular adenoma
   D. inflammatory polyp
   E. hyperplastic polyp

8. All of the following are true of thrombosed external hemorrhoids EXCEPT
   A. they present as sudden, painful swelling
   B. they may ulcerate and bleed
   C. they subside spontaneously within 24 hours
   D. they appear at the anal margin
   E. they respond rapidly to incision and enucleation of the clot

9. Horizontal spread of infection across the external sphincter can result in which type of anorectal abscess?
  A. ischiorectal
  B. perianal
  C. supralevator
  D. intersphincteric
  E. intermuscular

10. Treatment of paralytic ileus includes all of the following EXCEPT
  A. intravenous fluids
  B. nasogastric suction
  C. correction of electrolyte imbalance
  D. cessation of oral intake
  E. early operation

Questions 11 through 13

A 40-year-old female presents with upper abdominal pain and hyperamylasemia.

11. Disorders associated with hyperamylasemia include all of the following EXCEPT
  A. acute pancreatitis
  B. pernicious anemia
  C. perforated peptic ulcer
  D. ruptured aortic aneurysm
  E. parotiditis

12. Indications for surgery may include all of the following EXCEPT
  A. uncertainty of diagnosis
  B. pancreatic sepsis
  C. an amylase greater than 1000 units
  D. to correct associated biliary tract disease
  E. for progressive clinical deterioration

13. The patient is initially treated without surgery but 10 days later develops leukocytosis, fever, and increasing abdominal pain. A CT scan is obtained (Figure 3.2). Treatment may include all of the following EXCEPT
    A. antibiotic therapy
    B. external drainage
    C. debridement of necrotic pancreatic material
    D. near total pancreatectomy
    E. open packing

Questions 14 through 27

14. Common characteristics of small bowel obstruction include all of the following EXCEPT
    A. ascites
    B. frequent progression to strangulation
    C. failure to pass flatus
    D. distention
    E. vomiting

15. All of the following statements are true of diffuse esophageal spasm EXCEPT
    A. chest pain is frequently seen
    B. high amplitude esophageal contractions are present
    C. it is best diagnosed with barium esophogram
    D. usual surgical treatment is long esophagomyotomy
    E. most patients do not have significant coronary artery disease

16. All of the following statements are true of esophageal carcinoma EXCEPT
    A. operation is frequently curative
    B. squamous cell tumor is the most frequent histology
    C. patients usually die within one year of diagnosis
    D. patients can have intestinal continuity reestablished using the stomach after esophageal resection
    E. patients often require a pyloroplasty with operation

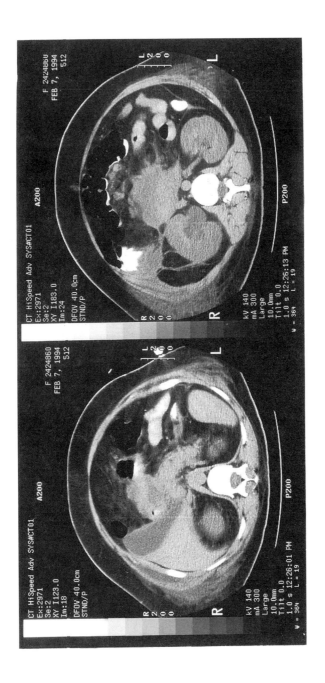

Figure 3.2

42

17. Gastroesophageal reflux is BEST diagnosed with
    A. radiography
    B. 24-hour pH monitoring of lower esophagus
    C. esophagoscopy
    D. documentation of a decrease in esophageal pH after HCl is placed in the stomach
    E. acid-clearing swallowing test

18. The risk of esophageal cancer increases with all of the following EXCEPT
    A. alcohol ingestion
    B. smoking
    C. chronic ingestion of hot beverages
    D. aflatoxin
    E. poor oral hygiene

19. Achalasia is associated with all of the following EXCEPT
    A. Chagas' disease in South America
    B. dysphasia
    C. weight loss
    D. relaxation of the lower esophageal sphincter with swallowing
    E. aspiration pneumonia, which may cause lung abscesses

20. Which of the following statements BEST describes a sliding (type I) hiatal hernia?
    A. it is a rare radiologic diagnosis
    B. it is usually associated with symptoms of gastroesophageal reflux
    C. it is an actual defect in the endoabdominal fascia
    D. an antireflux procedure should be recommended when the diagnosis is made
    E. the intra-abdominal segment of the esophagus below the insertion of the phrenoesophageal membrane is often of normal length

21. The treatment of an esophageal burn with a caustic agent may include all of the following EXCEPT
    A. expeditious administration of an antidote
    B. induction of vomiting
    C. steroids and antibiotics
    D. bougienage
    E. gastrectomy

22. The MOST important factor determining survival after perforation of the thoracic esophagus is the
    A. time interval between perforation and operation
    B. amount of associated bleeding
    C. etiology of the perforation
    D. use of a gastric fundus patch
    E. site of the perforation

23. All of the following substances are irritating to the peritoneum EXCEPT
    A. bile
    B. meconium
    C. blood
    D. gastric content
    E. pus

24. Nonsurgical causes of abdominal pain include all of the following EXCEPT
    A. pneumonia
    B. diabetic ketoacidosis
    C. acute salpingitis
    D. head trauma
    E. myocardial infarction

25. Gastric acid secretion is stimulated by all of the following EXCEPT
    A. sight of food
    B. presence of food in the stomach
    C. fat in the duodenum
    D. gastrin
    E. histamine

26. Paraesophageal (type II) hernias differ from sliding (type I) hernias in all of the following ways EXCEPT
   A. they usually require surgical repair to prevent incarceration and strangulation
   B. the phrenoesophageal membrane is intact
   C. although they may be asymptomatic, they usually progress to symptomatic complications
   D. large portions of the stomach—even the entire stomach—may become intrathoracic
   E. gastric volvulus may occur

27. Which of the following statements MOST accurately applies to the Zollinger–Ellison syndrome?
   A. 75% of patients will have multiple endocrine neoplasia type I
   B. requires total gastrectomy
   C. patients have an increase in gastrin with secretin stimulation
   D. patients usually have a basal acid secretion of less than 15 mEq/hr
   E. spontaneous resolution of the gastrinoma associated with the disease is common

Questions 28 through 30

A 74-year-old female presents with over 500 cc of hematemesis. Her abdominal exam is unremarkable.

28. After evaluation and stabilization, the BEST initial diagnostic test would be
   A. upper GI series
   B. esophagogastroduodenoscopy
   C. celiac axis arteriogram
   D. CT scan with oral and IV contrast
   E. gastric acid analysis

29. The LEAST likely cause of bleeding in this patient would be
   A. carcinoma
   B. duodenal ulcer
   C. esophageal varices
   D. gastric ulcer
   E. hemorrhagic gastritis

30. At endoscopy, a posterior duodenal ulcer is seen to be actively
bleeding. When it cannot be controlled endoscopically, surgery is
elected. The operation would include all of the following EXCEPT
   A. duodenotomy
   B. direct suture of bleeding point
   C. definitive ulcer operation, including vagotomy
   D. midline incision
   E. proximal anterior gastrotomy to rule out an associated Mal-
   lory–Weiss tear

Questions 31 through 47

31. Complications of truncal vagotomy and pyloroplasty include all
of the following EXCEPT
   A. dumping syndrome
   B. recurrent ulcer
   C. diarrhea
   D. alkaline reflux gastritis
   E. steatorrhea

32. Gastric polyps
   A. are most commonly adenomatous
   B. require gastrotomy and removal if greater than 2 cm and are
   pedunculated
   C. are rarely multiple
   D. are clearly premalignant
   E. are more frequent in achlorhydric patients

33. Mechanisms that may be important in the development of erosive
gastritis include all of the following EXCEPT
   A. local ischemia
   B. disruption of the mucosal barrier
   C. gastric acidity
   D. local increase of secretin
   E. availability of energy substrates

34. Vascular compression of the duodenum resulting in obstruction
   A. is present primarily in patients who are overweight
   B. should be given a trial of conservative management
   C. is common in pediatric patients

D. is best diagnosed by identifying a "double bubble" sign on abdominal x-ray

E. includes as medical therapy lying in the supine position after meals

35. Conditions associated with gastric cancer include all of the following EXCEPT

A. higher socioeconomic groups

B. pernicious anemia

C. chronic atrophic gastritis

D. adenomatous polyps

E. a high intake of dietary nitrates

36. In the treatment of gastric cancer, all of the following are true EXCEPT

A. five-year survival rates in the United States continue to be between 10% and 25%

B. total gastrectomy is mandated in most patients

C. lymph node involvement is associated with a poorer prognosis

D. palliative resection is frequently helpful with advanced disease

E. finding early disease at the time of operation is associated with a better prognosis

37. Patients with morbid obesity have an increased incidence of all of the following EXCEPT

A. gastric carcinoma

B. diabetes

C. stroke

D. gallbladder disease

E. joint deterioration

38. All of the following statements are true about patients with carcinoid tumors EXCEPT

A. they often have evidence of serotonin production

B. tumor growth is often slow

C. the majority have carcinoid syndrome

D. they have a much better prognosis if the tumors are less than 2 cm

E. the combination of streptozotocin and 5-fluorouracil can often result in objective response

39. All of the following contribute to malabsorption following truncal vagotomy and antrectomy EXCEPT

    A. increased rate of gastric emptying

    B. poor mixing of pancreatic secretions and bile salts with food

    C. increased release of secretin and cholecystokinin (CCK)

    D. decreased small intestinal transit time

    E. malabsorption of fat and carbohydrates

40. The treatment of choice for complete small bowel obstruction due to radiation-injured bowel is

    A. bypass of the diseased bowel

    B. resection of the diseased bowel

    C. multiple stricturoplasties

    D. long-term hyperalimentation

    E. high-dose steroids and sulfasalazine

41. A 20-year-old male with rebound tenderness in the right lower quadrant, fever, and a normal white blood cell count should generally be managed with

    A. intravenous antibiotics and nasogastric suction

    B. 24-hour observation

    C. exploratory laparotomy through a right lower quadrant incision

    D. exploratory laparotomy through a lower midline incision

    E. colonoscopy and identification of the appendiceal os

42. Indications for *emergency* operation for diverticulitis or diverticulosis include all of the following EXCEPT

    A. perforation

    B. fistula

    C. bleeding

    D. repeated attacks

    E. obstruction

43. The MOST likely diagnosis in an elderly patient with abdominal pain and colonoscopic findings of patchy mucosal ulceration at the splenic flexure is

    A. Crohn's colitis

    B. ischemic colitis

    C. diverticulitis

D. ulcerative colitis

E. lymphogranuloma venereum

44. Patients with right-sided colon cancer are more likely than patients with left-sided cancer to

A. have obstructive signs

B. show bright red blood in stools

C. present with anemia

D. have constipation

E. have lower abdominal pain

45. All of the following statements about ulcerative colitis are true EXCEPT

A. the disease is generally confined to the mucosa and submucosa of the colon

B. it almost always involves the rectum

C. corticosteroids and sulfasalazine are well accepted medical therapies

D. the surgical treatment of choice is total colectomy and ileoproctostomy

E. once the disease has been present over ten years, the risk of cancer increases dramatically

46. All of the following statements are true of anal fissure EXCEPT

A. it is often associated with constipation

B. pain during and after defecation is typical

C. the fissure is usually anterior

D. the lesion is commonly seen in Crohn's disease

E. division of the lower half of the internal sphincter is usually curative

47. The line of division between the right and left lobes of the liver is

A. the plane of the falciform ligament

B. a plane connecting the gallbladder fossa and the inferior vena cava

C. a plane from the fissure of the ligamentum teres to the diaphragmatic hiatus of the vena cava

D. at the caudate lobe

E. between segments II and VI

Questions 48 through 50

A 45-year-old male presents with symptomatic cholelithiasis and chooses to undergo laparoscopic cholecystectomy.

48. Advantages of laparoscopic versus open cholecystectomy include all of the following EXCEPT
    A. less risk of bile duct injury
    B. reduced hospitalization
    C. decreased pain
    D. reduced ileus
    E. improved cosmesis

49. The patient is discharged to home the day following surgery. Eight days after surgery, the patient presents with abdominal distention, vomiting, and mild right upper quadrant tenderness without peritoneal signs. The patient is afebrile and has a normal white blood cell count and a bilirubin of 1.5. The CT scan in Figure 3.3 is obtained. The MOST likely diagnosis is
    A. subhepatic abscess
    B. perforation of duodenal ulcer
    C. postoperative hemorrhage
    D. bile leak
    E. bile duct transection

50. Which of the following would be the most appropriate therapy for this patient?
    A. percutaneous drainage of fluid collection
    B. endoscopic retrograde cholangiography and nasobiliary stenting
    C. both A and B
    D. relaparoscopy and treatment
    E. exploratory laparotomy and treatment

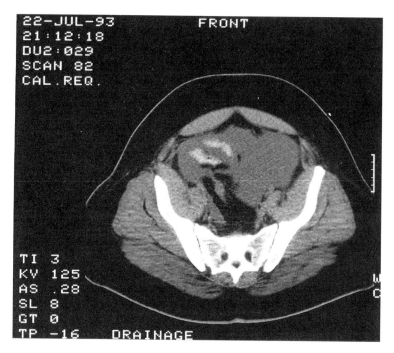

Figure 3.3

Questions 51 through 65

51. All of the following statements are true of hepatocellular carcinoma EXCEPT
    A. it is often associated with alpha-fetoprotein
    B. a long duration of symptoms is usually seen
    C. it is often hypervascular on arteriogram
    D. liver resection is the best current treatment
    E. it is at increased risk of developing in patients with cirrhosis

52. All of the following statements are true of hemobilia EXCEPT
   A. the most common cause is trauma
   B. the diagnosis is suggested with the triad of gastrointestinal bleeding, right upper quadrant pain, and jaundice
   C. the most accurate diagnostic procedure is computed tomography
   D. treatment may include ligation of the common hepatic artery
   E. if bleeding is minor, it is best managed expectantly

53. Treatment of chronic ascites may include all of the following EXCEPT
   A. dietary sodium restriction
   B. aldosterone antagonists
   C. loop diuretics
   D. potassium supplementation
   E. peritoneovenous shunting

54. Transjugular intrahepatic portasystemic shunt (TIPS) can be used for the treatment of acute bleeding from esophageal varices due to portal hypertension. Advantages of the TIPS compared to a portacaval shunt include all of the following EXCEPT
   A. less surgical morbidity
   B. less encephalopathy
   C. subsequent transplant less difficult
   D. less mortality in patients with minimal hepatic reserve
   E. greater decrease in the portasystemic pressure gradient

55. Complications of peritoneovenous shunting may include all of the following EXCEPT
   A. coagulopathy
   B. infection
   C. renal failure
   D. superior vena caval thrombosis
   E. pulmonary edema

56. Posttransfusion hepatitis is MOST often due to
   A. hepatitis A
   B. hepatitis B
   C. non-A, non-B virus (hepatitis C)

    D.   delta-associated virus

    E.   Epstein–Barr virus

57. Choledocholithiasis in a patient who previously had cholecystectomy is BEST treated with

    A.   endoscopic sphincterotomy

    B.   choledochoduodenostomy

    C.   dissolution with mono-octanoin

    D.   choledochojejunostomy

    E.   open common bile duct exploration with stone removal

58. In the treatment of acute cholecystitis, most patients are BEST served with

    A.   early cholecystectomy (within 3 days of onset of symptoms)

    B.   IV antibiotics and cholecystectomy in 6 to 8 weeks

    C.   percutaneous drainage of the gallbladder

    D.   endoscopic sphincterotomy

    E.   cholecystostomy

59. Factors important in the formation of gallstones include all of the following EXCEPT

    A.   cholesterol saturation of bile

    B.   gallbladder dysmotility

    C.   nucleating agents

    D.   obesity

    E.   the size of the micelles

60. Management of cholangitis may include all of the following EXCEPT

    A.   decompression of the common bile duct

    B.   cholecystostomy

    C.   IV antibiotics

    D.   correct underlying cause

    E.   percutaneous transhepatic cholangiography

61. Carcinoma of the gallbladder is

    A.   associated with a good prognosis

    B.   most commonly metastatic to the lung

    C.   rarely associated with jaundice

    D.   usually not diagnosed preoperatively

    E.   best treated with radiation and chemotherapy

62. Factors that are associated with the development of acute pancreatitis include all of the following EXCEPT

    A. alcohol
    B. gallstones
    C. celiac sprue
    D. hyperlipidemia
    E. pancreatic divisum

63. Complications of untreated pancreatic pseudocysts include all of the following EXCEPT

    A. gastrointestinal obstruction
    B. pancreatic necrosis
    C. free rupture
    D. abscess
    E. intracystic hemorrhage

64. Common presenting conditions in patients with pancreatic carcinoma include all of the following EXCEPT

    A. esophageal varices
    B. jaundice
    C. weight loss
    D. palpable gallbladder
    E. abdominal pain

65. The superior and medial structure used in an inguinal hernia repair is the

    A. inguinal ligament
    B. iliopubic tract
    C. transversus abdominis aponeurotic arch
    D. lacunar ligament
    E. rectus sheath

Questions 66 through 69

Three months after laparoscopic cholecystectomy for symptomatic cholelithiasis, a middle-aged woman presented with recurrent right upper quadrant pain and jaundice. Her transhepatic cholangiogram is shown in Figure 3.4.

66. The diagnosis is
    A. stricture of the common bile duct
    B. cancer of the head of the pancreas
    C. choledocholithiasis
    D. common duct stricture due to pancreatitis
    E. ampullary cancer

67. If the diagnosis is choledocholithiasis, all of the following suggest that the origin of stones may have been the gallbladder EXCEPT
    A. the consistency of the stones is soft and mudlike
    B. the prior cholecystectomy specimen contained a single multifaceted stone
    C. the stones are of mixed type and firm
    D. the symptoms precipitating the cholecystectomy were not improved following surgery
    E. both the cystic duct and the common duct were noted to be enlarged at the prior operation

68. If the diagnosis is pancreatic cancer, all of the following are true EXCEPT
    A. the disease is often asymptomatic in early stages
    B. it was likely present, but not noted, at the prior operation
    C. the radiologic picture is characterized by Figure 3.4
    D. the radiologic picture usually shows a tapering of the common duct in the area of the head of the pancreas
    E. the prognosis is generally less favorable than ampullary cancer

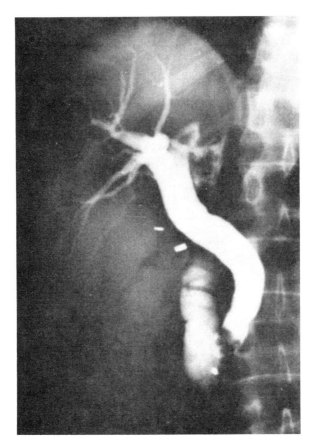

Figure 3.4

69. If the diagnosis is choledocholithiasis, all of the following would be acceptable treatments EXCEPT

    A. endoscopic sphincterotomy and stone extraction

    B. percutaneous stone extraction

    C. common duct exploration, stone removal and T-tube placement

    D. operative removal of stones and choledochoduodenostomy

    E. operative removal of stones and Roux-en-Y choledochojejunostomy

Abdominal Surgery

Answers and Comments

1. **(D)** Tenderness in the right lower quadrant is the most important finding in acute appendicitis, although all diagnostic tests are fallible. Vomiting, fever, and leukocytosis are often but not always present. Rovsing's sign, or pain in the right lower quadrant when palpation is done in the left lower quadrant, is a manifestation of referred rebound tenderness and can be helpful in supporting a diagnosis of appendicitis. (**Ref. 1,** p. 887; **Ref. 3,** p. 1317; **Ref. 4,** p. 193)

2. **(C)** Paralytic ileus shows a uniform distribution of gas in the stomach, small bowel, and colon on abdominal x-ray. Radiographs of patients with small bowel obstruction show no gas in the colon. Patients with distal colon obstruction and an incompetent ileocecal valve can appear similar to a paralytic ileus and is best differentiated with a contrast agent enema. Peritonitis is associated with paralytic ileus. Adhesions, annular pancreas, volvulus, and intussusception are all etiologies of bowel obstruction. (**Ref. 1,** p. 840; **Ref. 3,** p. 1084)

3. **(B)** Hypersplenism associated with portal hypertension secondary to cirrhosis seldom requires splenectomy. Isolated splenic injuries may be treated nonoperatively but usually require

splenectomy when severe and associated with other sources of hemorrhage. The remaining conditions commonly require splenectomy. (**Ref. 3,** pp. 1447–1448; **Ref. 4,** p. 306)

4. **(D)** The primary indication for surgery in Crohn's disease is partial intestinal obstruction produced by the fibrotic response to the inflammatory process of the disease. Enterocutaneous fistula and the associated intra-abdominal abscess and abdominal mass are another common indication for surgery. Internal fistulae often do not require surgery, and gastrointestinal bleeding is rarely an indication for surgery in small intestinal Crohn's disease. (**Ref. 3,** p. 1249; **Ref. 4,** p. 204)

5. **(D)** The ileum is the narrowest portion of the intestines and thus the most frequent site of gallstone ileus. (**Ref. 3,** p. 1394; **Ref. 4,** p. 242)

6. **(E)** The most important aspect to creating a trouble-free ileostomy is to "mature" the ileostomy as described by Brooke. This involves bringing approximately 5 cm of ileum above the level of the skin and folding back the tip so the ileostomy protrudes 2 to 3 cm above the skin. Eversion of the ileostomy to expose only mucosa prevents serositis that is seen when the serosa is exposed. (**Ref. 1,** p. 935; **Ref. 3,** p. 494)

7. **(A)** Approximately 40% of villous adenomas show malignant change. Adenomas have a 5% chance of showing malignant change, while the other polyps have little or no increase in malignant potential. (**Ref. 3,** p. 1264; **Ref. 4,** p. 216)

8. **(C)** External hemorrhoids present as sudden painful swelling at the anal margin. They may cause overlying skin necrosis, resulting in skin ulceration and hemorrhoidal bleeding. The natural history of thrombosed external hemorrhoids is to have pain for several days that gradually subsides spontaneously. Response to surgery is rapid. (**Ref. 1,** p. 962–963; **Ref. 3,** p. 1302)

9. **(A)** Anorectal abscesses begin in the anal glands that reside between internal and external sphincters and open into the rectum at the dentate line. An intersphincteric abscess is confined to the primary site. Proximal vertical spread gives an intermuscular ab-

scess or a supralevator abscess if it crosses the longitudinal muscle above the levator muscle group. Perianal abscess is the result of distal vertical spread to the anal margin. An ischiorectal abscess will result from the spread of infection across the internal and external sphincter into the ischiorectal fossa. (**Ref. 1,** p. 965; **Ref. 3,** p. 1300)

10. **(E)** The standard treatment of ileus is to stop all oral intake, give intravenous fluid, institute nasogastric suction, and correct any electrolyte imbalances. Operative therapy is usually not necessary. (**Ref. 1,** pp. 835–836; **Ref. 2,** p. 1031)

11. **(B)** Hyperamylasemia is most commonly seen with pancreatic disorders. However, there is a high false-positive and false-negative rate. In an acute hospital setting, nearly one-third of elevations in amylase are unrelated to the pancreas. A multitude of disorders cause hyperamylasemia. Some common ones include: perforated peptic ulcer, ruptured abdominal aortic aneurysm, intestinal obstruction, and parotiditis. Pernicious anemia is not associated with hyperamylasemia. (**Ref. 1,** p. 1082)

12. **(C)** In patients with suspected acute pancreatitis, if the diagnosis is not firm, or if there is clinical deterioration despite optimum support, exploratory laparotomy may be indicated to exclude the presence of a surgically correctable cause. Pancreatic abscess formation can develop in necrotic pancreatic tissue and require drainage. Biliary pancreatitis usually resolves quickly and cholecystectomy can be performed within 5 to 7 days. The degree of amylasemia is not a reliable predictor of the severity of the pancreatitis or whether surgery should be done. (**Ref. 1,** pp. 1086–1087; **Ref. 2,** pp. 1408–1409)

13. **(D)** Figure 3.2 shows a 5-cm pancreatic abscess. Treatment includes antibiotic therapy and drainage. Infected necrotic pancreatic material often requires operative debridement. In severe cases, open packing of the abscess allows multiple packing changes until the necrotic material is cleared and the infection controlled. Anatomic pancreatectomy should not be perfomed in patients with pancreatic abscess. (**Ref. 1,** p. 1087; **Ref. 2,** pp. 1410–1412)

14. (A)   The abdomen is usually somewhat distended with small bowel obstruction. The abdominal distention associated with small bowel obstruction can be differentiated from that of ascites with careful physical examination. Vomiting, failure to pass flatus, and frequent progression to strangulation are some of the characteristics of small bowel obstruction. (**Ref. 1,** pp. 835–836; **Ref. 4,** p. 199)

15. (C)   Esophageal manometry is the best test to diagnose diffuse esophageal spasm. These patients have high amplitude simultaneous esophageal contractions that can produce chest pain. Patients are often diagnosed after a normal coronary arteriogram. If the patient comes to operation, long esophagomyotomy is most frequently used. (**Ref. 1,** p. 670; **Ref. 3,** p. 1112)

16. (A)   In the vast majority of patients with esophageal carcinoma, local tumor invasion or distant metastases preclude cure, and most patients die within a year. Squamous cell tumor is the most frequent histology, although adenocarcinomas have been increasing in incidence in recent years. The stomach is the most common portion of the GI tract to establish continuity after esophageal resection. (**Ref. 1,** pp. 690–691; **Ref. 3,** p. 1140; **Ref. 4,** p. 172)

17. (B)   Prolonged monitoring of the pH in the lower esophagus over a 24-hour period is the most precise and useful quantitative method for diagnosing gastroesophageal reflux. (**Ref. 1,** p. 709; **Ref. 3,** p. 1107)

18. (D)   Factors that increase the risk of esophageal cancer include alcohol ingestion, smoking, zinc, nitrosamines, malnutrition, anemia, poor oral hygiene, previous gastric surgery, and chronic ingestion of hot foods or beverages. Aflatoxin increases the risk of hepatocellular carcinoma. (**Ref. 1,** pp. 690–691; **Ref. 3,** p. 1138)

19. (D)   The manometric criteria of achalasia are failure of the lower esophageal sphincter to relax reflexively when swallowing and lack of progressive peristalsis through the length of the esophagus. Dysphasia, weight loss, and aspiration pneumonia with secondary lung abscesses are also possible complications of achalasia. Chagas' disease can be the etiology for acquired achalasia if patients are from an endemic area. (**Ref. 1,** pp. 666, 4, 170)

20. (E) A hiatal hernia is the herniation of an abdominal organ, usually the stomach, through the esophageal hiatus of the diaphragm. With a sliding hiatal hernia, the endoabdominal fascia remains intact but stretches, allowing a portion of the stomach to slide above the diaphragm. The endoabdominal fascia defines the boundary of the abdomen, and the intra-abdominal segment of the esophagus is often of normal length, even though it is located above the diaphragm. Sliding hernias are usually not associated with symptoms unless gastroesophageal reflux is also present. A sliding hiatal hernia is commonly seen on upper GI series and endoscopy. (**Ref. 1,** pp. 706–707; **Ref. 3,** p. 1119)

21. (B) Induced vomiting and gastric lavage are contraindicated after caustic ingestion because of the danger of compounding the original injury. Acid or alkaline antidotes may be helpful if used in the first few minutes. Steroids with antibiotics, as well as bougienage, are standard treatments. Necrosis of the stomach may require gastrectomy. (**Ref. 1,** p. 716–717; **Ref. 4,** p. 173)

22. (A) Survival following perforation of the thoracic esophagus varies directly with the time interval between perforation and operation. Mortality is 10% to 15% in patients treated within 24 hours of injury, but increases to 50% if delay is 24 hours or greater. Principles of surgery include control of the site of perforation and drainage. (**Ref. 1,** p. 703; **Ref. 4,** p. 173)

23. (C) Blood is not an irritating substance in the peritoneum. Infection is the most common cause of peritonitis. Chemical peritonitis is a sterile or nearly sterile substance that irritates the peritoneum, usually due to body fluids such as bile, meconium, urine, or gastric content. (**Ref. 1,** pp. 745–746; **Ref. 3,** pp. 1475–1476)

24. (D) Common causes of abdominal pain not requiring operation for treatment include: myocardial infarction, pneumonia, pulmonary infarction, pancreatitis, gastroenteritis, hepatitis, diabetic ketoacidosis, hyperlipidemia, rectus muscle hematoma, peripheral neuralgia, pyelonephritis, acute salpingitis, and sickle cell crisis. Head trauma may have associated abdominal trauma but is not in itself a cause of abdominal pain. (**Ref. 1,** p. 738; **Ref. 3,** p. 1064)

25. (C) The sight or smell of food results in a vagus-mediated increase in gastric secretion (cephalic phase). Food in the stomach (gastric phase) results in gastrin release and increased gastric secretions. In the proper neurohormonal milieu, histamine is released from stores within the gastric mucosa and stimulates acid secretion. Gastric acid secretion is inhibited by the presence of acid, fat, or hyperosmotic solutions in the duodenum. (**Ref. 1,** p. 758; **Ref. 3,** p. 1163)

26. (B) Paraesophageal hernias are an indication for surgery, as there is a defect in the phrenoesophageal ligament and incarceration and strangulation of abdominal organs can occur. Gastric volvulus is associated with paraesophageal hernias. (**Ref. 1,** pp. 706–707; **Ref. 2,** p. 1111)

27. (C) The hypergastrinemia seen in Zollinger–Ellison syndrome is augmented by secretin infusion. Only 25% of patients have a type I multiple endocrine neoplasia. Basal secretion of acid is usually greater than 15 mEq/hr, and many patients can be treated medically and do not require gastrectomy. Spontaneous resolution of the tumor is rare. (**Ref. 1,** pp. 771–772; **Ref. 3,** p. 1170; **Ref. 4,** pp. 182, 255)

28. (B) Endoscopy is the most important test because it can localize the site of the upper GI bleeding, and often treatment can be provided via the endoscope. Roentgenograms may show an ulcer or varices but cannot identify the site of bleeding. An arteriogram may identify the site of bleeding and allow the local infusion of vasopressors to control bleeding, but it is reserved for patients who cannot be controlled endoscopically. CT scan and gastric acid analysis have no place in the diagnosis of acute upper GI bleeding. (**Ref. 1,** p. 768; **Ref. 2,** p. 1032)

29. (A) The most common cause of significant upper GI bleeding in descending order of occurrence are: duodenal ulcer, hemorrhagic gastritis, esophageal varices, and gastric ulcer. Less common causes of upper GI bleeding include Mallory–Weiss tear, esophagitis, and carcinoma. (**Ref. 1,** p. 768; **Ref. 2,** p. 1032)

30. (E) The primary goal of the operation is to control the bleeding. This is done by direct suturing of the bleeding point. Access to the bleeding site is via an anterior duodenotomy. The midline incision is most appropriate in an emergency situation because it can be performed more quickly. A definitive ulcer operation which will include vagotomy is then performed if the patient is stable. The endoscopy should exclude a Mallory–Weiss tear, and anterior gastrostomy is not generally required. (**Ref. 1,** pp. 768–769; **Ref. 2,** p. 1033)

31. **(E)** Common complications after truncal vagotomy and pyloroplasty include dumping syndrome, recurrent ulcer, diarrhea, gastroparesis, and alkaline reflux gastritis. Steatorrhea is occasionally seen after Billroth II gastrectomy and probably results from bypass of the duodenum. (**Ref. 1,** pp. 778–780; **Ref. 4,** p. 181)

32. **(E)** Gastric polyps are usually hyperplastic, rather than adenomatous, and can be multiple. Pedunculated polyps can usually be safely removed endoscopically, even if they are greater than 2 cm. There is little evidence that the hyperplastic polyp itself is premalignant. Adenomatous polyps are more frequently seen in achlorhydria patients. (**Ref. 1,** p. 789; **Ref. 3,** pp. 1178–1179; **Ref. 4,** p. 186)

33. **(D)** Experimental evidence has implicated all of these as a mechanism of development of erosive gastritis except local increase of secretin. Secretin is released in the duodenum in response to increased duodenal acid. (**Ref. 1,** pp. 798–799; **Ref. 3,** p. 1173)

34. **(B)** Vascular compression of the duodenum resulting in obstruction is a rare disease and, when present, is often seen in patients who have lost weight. The disease can be diagnosed with barium studies of the duodenum, occasionally supplemented with biplanar aortography. A trial of conservative management, including hyperalimentation and placement of the patient in a prone or left-lateral decubitus position after meals, is indicated. (**Ref. 1,** p. 811)

35. **(A)** Patients with achlorhydria (pernicious anemia and chronic atrophic gastritis) are at increased risk of developing gastric cancer. Adenomatous gastric polyps can be precursors of cancer, and there is some evidence implicating the formation of nitrosamines

from nitrates in the etiology of gastric cancer. The incidence of gastric cancer is greater in lower socioeconomic groups. (**Ref. 1,** p. 815; **Ref. 3,** p. 1177)

36. **(B)** In general, resection for the usual distal gastric cancer should include a subtotal gastrectomy. Improved survival rates have not been definitely demonstrated with total gastrectomy. The five-year survival rate in patients with gastric cancer is 10% to 25%. Early gastric cancer improves prognosis, while prognosis is worse if lymph node involvement is present. Patients with advanced gastric cancer will be more comfortable and may live longer following palliative resection. (**Ref. 1,** pp. 820–821; **Ref. 3,** p. 1178)

37. **(A)** Morbidly obese patients do not have an increased risk of developing gastric carcinoma. However, there is a clear correlation between excess weight and the other factors listed. (**Ref. 1,** pp. 851–852; **Ref. 3,** p. 1181)

38. **(C)** Only about 7% of patients with carcinoid tumors have carcinoid syndrome. Approximately 50% of patients with carcinoid tumors of gastrointestinal origin have evidence of serotonin production. Prognosis is better for those patients with tumors less than 2 cm, and tumor growth is often slow. Streptozotocin and 5-fluorouracil are a useful drug combination in the treatment of advanced carcinoid tumors. (**Ref. 1,** pp. 871–872; **Ref. 3,** p. 1208)

39. **(C)** Rapid gastric emptying, decreased intestine transit time, poor mixing of pancreatic secretions and bile acids with food, as well as decreased glucose absorption, can all contribute to malabsorption after vagotomy and antrectomy. The release of secretin and CCK is usually diminished after truncal vagotomy. (**Ref. 1,** pp. 876)

40. **(B)** Surgical exploration is necessary in patients who have a complete obstruction due to radiation injury of the small bowel. When possible, resection of the diseased bowel is the treatment of choice. Where diseased bowel may not be safely removed, bypass is occasionally the best option. Stricturoplasties are contraindicated due to the risk of fistula formation. (**Ref. 1,** pp. 882–883; **Ref. 3,** p. 1251)

41. (C) In cases of suspected appendicitis, if clinical findings are at variance with the white blood cell count, clinical findings should take precedence. For presumed uncomplicated appendicitis, a right lower quadrant incision is preferred. (**Ref. 1,** p. 888; **Ref. 3,** p. 1317; **Ref. 4,** p. 193)

42. (D) Patients with repeated attacks of diverticulitis should undergo elective resection of the involved colon. The other indications are for complications of diverticulitis or diverticulosis that often require emergency surgery. (**Ref. 1,** pp. 916–917; **Ref. 3,** pp. 1256–1257)

43. (B) Ischemic colitis can occur anywhere in the colon, but the splenic flexure and descending colon are most vulnerable. The syndrome usually occurs in older patients; mild abdominal pain and bleeding of bright red blood are the most common symptoms. The mucosal surface shows edema, darkening, and patchy ulceration. (**Ref. 3,** pp. 1249–1250)

44. (C) Left-sided colon cancers present with rectal bleeding, altered bowel habits, obstructions, and lower abdominal pain. Right-sided cancers more commonly present with occult blood in the stool, anemia, dyspepsia, and upper abdominal pain. (**Ref. 1,** p. 946; **Ref. 3,** p. 1277; **Ref. 4,** pp. 216–217)

45. (D) The surgical treatment of ulcerative colitis requires removal of the colon and rectal mucosa to obtain a definitive cure. This can be accomplished with total proctocolectomy and permanent ileostomy. New approaches such as proctocolectomy with colo-anal anastomosis or total colectomy, mucosal proctectomy, and ileoanal anastomosis can cure the disease yet retain anal continence. Surgical treatment with total colectomy and ileoproctostomy is usually not indicated because the risk of proctitis and development of carcinoma remains. The other statements about ulcerative colitis are true. (**Ref. 1,** p. 935; **Ref. 3,** pp. 1238–1243; **Ref. 4,** pp. 220–222)

46. (C) Anal fissure is most often situated posteriorly. It is usually associated with constipation, and pain after defecation is typical. It is important to remember Crohn's disease in the differential diagnosis to allow optimum treatment. Lateral internal sphincterotomy is nearly always curative. (**Ref. 1,** pp. 967–968; **Ref. 3,** p. 1303; **Ref. 4,** pp. 228–229)

47. (B)   A plane connecting the gallbladder fossa and the inferior vena cava separate the right and left lobes of the liver. The falciform ligament divides the left lobe of the liver into medial and lateral segments. Most of the caudate lobe is in the left lobe of the liver, but it extends into the anatomic right lobe. In the subsegmental anatomy of the liver as defined by Couinaud, the line of division is between segment IV in the left lobe and segments V and VIII in the right lobe. (**Ref. 1,** pp. 977–978; **Ref. 3,** p. 1327)

48. (A)   The risk of bile duct injury with open cholecystectomy is approximately 0.2 percent. Although the incidence of this complication during laparoscopic cholecystectomy is still unknown, bile duct injury probably occurs more frequently than during open cholecystectomy. Laparoscopic cholecystectomy clearly reduces hospitalization, decreases pain, reduces ileus, and improves cosmesis compared to open cholecystectomy. (**Ref. 1,** p. 1054)

49. (D)   All of the conditions listed would be in the differential diagnosis. The most likely diagnosis would be a bile leak from the cystic duct or bile duct. A subhepatic abscess would likely be associated with a fever and leukocytosis. A perforated ulcer generally has pronounced peritoneal signs. Postoperative hemorrhage usually manifests itself in the first two days postoperatively, and complete bile duct transection would likely be associated with greater hyperbilirubinemia.(**Ref. 2,** p. 1387)

50. (C)   Treatment includes percutaneous drainage of the bile leak to avoid secondary infection and ERCP to define the leak. If a cystic duct leak or a small bile duct leak is present, without compromise of the bile duct, a nasobiliary stent should be placed to decompress the bile duct as the leak seals. Relaparoscopy six days postop would be difficult due to immature fibrosis. Cystic duct leak can generally be treated without laparotomy. (**Ref. 2,** p. 1387)

51. (B)   The duration of symptoms is often surprisingly short. In one series, over 75% of patients had symptoms of less than six weeks' duration. Alpha-fetoprotein is present in over 50% of patients.

Liver resection is the only therapy that substantially prolongs survival. Risk factors for the development of hepatocellular carcinoma include hepatitis B, alcoholic cirrhosis, aflatoxin, hemochromatosis, alpha-antitrypsin deficiency, and blood group B. (**Ref. 1,** pp. 999–1000; **Ref. 3,** p. 1349; **Ref. 4,** p. 297)

52. **(C)** Usually the most accurate diagnostic procedure in cases of suspected hemobilia is hepatic arteriography. Trauma, often iatrogenic, is the most important etiologic factor. The classic signs and symptoms associated with hemobilia are gastrointestinal bleeding, right upper quadrant pain, and jaundice. Minor bleeding is best managed expectantly. Ligation of the common hepatic artery is a possible treatment. It rarely results in clinically evident hepatic ischemia due to abundant collateral blood supply. (**Ref. 1,** pp. 1012–1013)

53. **(D)** Patients taking potassium-sparing diuretics, such as aldosterone antagonists, should avoid potassium supplements. Dietary sodium restriction, aldosterone antagonists, loop diuretics, and peritoneovenous shunting are all established treatments for chronic ascites. (**Ref. 1,** p. 1031; **Ref. 3,** p. 1360)

54. **(E)** The transjugular intrahepatic portasystemic shunt reduces portal pressure and is usually successful in stopping bleeding from esophageal varices. The shunt can be placed percutaneously and thus has less surgical morbidity. The TIPS is a partial shunt and thus does not decrease the portasystemic pressure gradient as much as a portacaval shunt. Because some portal blood flow to the liver is maintained, the risk of encephalopathy and mortality in patients with minimal hepatic reserve is less. A portacaval shunt can compromise future liver transplant operations. (**Ref. 1,** pp. 1021–1023)

55. **(C)** Peritoneovenous shunting is associated with a rise in renal blood flow and a decrease in renin and aldosterone levels. The shunt can be effective in treating hepatorenal syndrome, which includes a functional renal failure. All patients develop a degree of coagulopathy that may necessitate discontinuance of the shunt. Infection is a serious complication, requiring removal of the shunt. Pulmonary edema can result from increased intravascular fluid, and the catheter can contribute to superior vena caval

thrombosis. The procedure is contraindicated in cases of established renal failure as the influx of ascitic fluid cannot be excreted. (**Ref. 1,** pp. 1031–1032)

56. **(C)** Posttransfusion hepatitis is most often due to hepatitis C. Hepatitis B and delta hepatitis are also principally transmitted by the parenteral route. Hepatitis A is usually transmitted by the fecal–oral route, and parenteral transmission is unusual. (**Ref. 1,** p. 1037; **Ref. 3,** p. 133)

57. **(A)** Choledocholithiasis is generally best treated by endoscopic sphincterotomy. Relative contraindications to sphincterotomy include distal common duct stricture, duodenal diverticula, coagulation disorders, and recent pancreatitis. Operative treatment is usually not necessary, and mono-octanoin dissolution is possible for some stones but requires 1 to 2 weeks of therapy. (**Ref. 1,** p. 1046; **Ref. 3,** p. 1393; **Ref. 4,** p. 241)

58. **(A)** Prospective trials show that the mortality rates for early and delayed surgery are equal, and the frequency and severity of postoperative complications are similar. Early cholecystectomy is preferred because it shortens hospital stay and reduces the time out of work. Percutaneous drainage can help avoid general anesthesia in high-risk patients. Cholecystostomy should be performed if cholecystectomy is not safe. Endoscopic sphincterotomy has no role in the treatment of acute cholecystitis. (**Ref. 1,** p. 1052; **Ref. 4,** p. 237)

59. **(E)** The etiology of gallstones is multifactorial. Cholesterol saturation of bile, stasis of bile within the gallbladder, and nucleating factors are important. Obesity, exogenous estrogen, truncal vagotomy, and pregnancy are other predisposing factors. (**Ref. 1,** p. 1057; **Ref. 3,** p. 1390; **Ref. 4,** p. 233)

60. **(B)** Cholecystostomy does not decompress the common bile duct adequately and should not be done for cholangitis. IV antibiotics are often effective in the treatment of mild cholangitis. Acute toxic cholangitis unresponsive to antibiotics requires decompression of the biliary duct system. After cholangitis resolves, diagnostic studies should be done and the underlying problem corrected. (**Ref. 1,** p. 1069; **Ref. 3,** p. 1399)

61. (D)   Carcinoma of the gallbladder presents similarly to benign gallbladder disease, and the diagnosis is seldom made preoperatively. Jaundice is often seen and is due to invasion or compression of the common bile duct. Metastatic spread is most common via lymphatics, either to pericholedochal nodes or to the liver. The prognosis is dismal; most survivors have surgery for what is presumed to be benign biliary disease. (**Ref. 1,** p. 1074; **Ref. 3,** p. 1403; **Ref. 4,** p. 238)

62. (C)   The two most common causes of acute pancreatitis are alcohol and gallstones. Miscellaneous factors associated with pancreatitis include hyperlipidemia and pancreatic divisum, ischemia, drugs, endoscopic retrograde pancreatography, trauma, viral disease, and hypercalcemia. (**Ref. 1,** p. 1081; **Ref. 3,** p. 1418; **Ref. 4,** pp. 247–248)

63. (B)   Complications of untreated pseudocysts include infection, gastrointestinal obstruction, rupture, and intracystic hemorrhage. Pancreatic necrosis can be a complication of acute pancreatitis but is usually not a result of pseudocysts. (**Ref. 1,** p. 1092; **Ref. 3,** p. 1428; **Ref. 4,** p. 251)

64. (A)   Common presenting symptoms in patients with pancreatic carcinoma include jaundice, weight loss, and abdominal or back pain. Some patients with jaundice will have a palpable gallbladder. Most patients with jaundice due to choledocholithiasis will not have a palpable gallbladder because the inflamed gallbladder is incapable of distending (Courvoisier's law). Esophageal varices are not a common presenting condition in patients with pancreatic carcinoma. (**Ref. 1,** p. 1096; **Ref. 3,** p. 1430; **Ref. 4,** p. 252)

65. (C)   The muscle of the transversus abdominis is replaced by a tendinous aponeurosis, which fuses with the internal oblique aponeurosis to form the rectus sheath. Lateral to the rectus sheath, the inferior free margin of the transversalis aponeurosis arches superiorly and medially to the internal inguinal ring and inguinal canal. This transversus abdominis aponeurotic arch forms a basic component of the anatomic repair of all inguinal hernias. (**Ref. 1,** p. 1140; **Ref. 3,** p. 1536)

66. **(C)** The x-ray picture shows common bile duct dilatation and multiple gallstones. The common bile duct is dilated down to the ampulla, and no strictures are evident. Pancreatic malignancies or pancreatitis show a stricture in the head of the pancreas. Common bile duct injuries after cholecystectomy are generally close to the insertion of the cystic duct. Ampullary cancer can cause dilatation, but is usually not associated with choledocholithiasis. (**Ref. 1**, p. 1045; **Ref. 3**, pp. 1392–1393)

67. **(A)** Stones that form in the common duct are usually soft, mud-like, and rounded. Stones from the gallbladder usually are of mixed type and firm. A multifaceted stone indicates the past presence of other gallstones as single gallstones are rounded. (**Ref. 1**, p. 1045)

68. **(C)** Figure 2.4 shows choledocholithiasis. Pancreatic cancer usually shows tapering of the common duct in the head of the pancreas and is not associated with gallstones. The five-year survival for resectable ampullary cancer is 3 to 5 times that of resectable pancreatic cancer. (**Ref. 1**, p. 1096; **Ref. 3**, p. 1432)

69. **(B)** Percutaneous stone extraction is usually done through an established bile drainage tract (T-tube tract). The choice of whether to perform a ductal drainage procedure connecting the duct to the duodenum or jejunum is usually decided at operation, depending upon the condition of the duct, ability to relieve the obstruction, and the cause of the ductal stones. Endoscopic sphincterotomy and stone extraction are an accepted alternative and especially attractive in patients at high risk for surgery. (**Ref. 1**, pp. 1046–1047; **Ref. 3**, p. 1392)

4

Breast and Endocrine Surgery

Debra G. Koivunen
Paul Yazdi

DIRECTIONS (Questions 1 through 40): Each of the questions or incomplete statements below is followed by five suggested answers or completions. Select the ONE that is best in each case.

1. All of the following are associated with an increased risk of breast cancer EXCEPT
   - A. dietary consumption of fat
   - B. history of breast cancer in first-degree maternal relatives
   - C. age over 35
   - D. early first pregnancy
   - E. infertility

2. The MOST frequent histologic type of breast carcinoma is
   - A. infiltrating papillary carcinoma
   - B. infiltrating ductal carcinoma
   - C. infiltrating lobular carcinoma
   - D. colloid carcinoma
   - E. medullary carcinoma

3. The correct sequence of events for the metabolism of iodine and synthesis of thyroid hormone is
   A. trapping, organification, coupling, release, oxidation
   B. oxidation, trapping, coupling, organification, release
   C. coupling, organification, trapping, oxidation, release
   D. trapping, oxidation, organification, coupling, release
   E. trapping, coupling, oxidation, release, organification

4. The MOST frequent variety of thyroid cancer is
   A. follicular carcinoma
   B. papillary carcinoma
   C. anaplastic carcinoma
   D. Hashimoto's associated lymphoma
   E. medullary carcinoma

5. Hypoparathyroidism in adults is MOST commonly a result of
   A. development of antiparathyroid antibodies (Schmidt's syndrome)
   B. prior neck surgery
   C. ^{131}I therapy
   D. lack of parathyroid-stimulating factor (PSF) from the pituitary
   E. congenital absence of parathyroid glands (DiGeorge's syndrome)

6. Secretion of insulin by the pancreas is controlled primarily by
   A. the vagus nerves
   B. secretin
   C. glucagon
   D. the blood sugar level
   E. ingestion of a meal

7. The precursor of all adrenal steroids is
   A. phenylalanine
   B. tyrosine
   C. arachidonic acid
   D. cholesterol
   E. none of the above

8. Hormones secreted by the anterior pituitary include all of the following EXCEPT
   A. follicle-stimulating hormone
   B. oxytocin
   C. adrenocortical trophic hormone
   D. growth hormone
   E. prolactin

9. Mammographic lesions that are strongly associated with malignancy include all of the following EXCEPT
   A. large and coarse calcifications
   B. thickened epidermis
   C. poorly defined mass lesions
   D. fine stippled calcifications
   E. increased density

10. Acute mastitis MOST commonly occurs at or during
    A. birth
    B. puberty
    C. pregnancy
    D. lactation
    E. blunt trauma to the breast

11. All of the following statements concerning nipple discharges are true EXCEPT
    A. they may be caused by multiple lesions
    B. when bloody, the discharge is due to a malignancy 70% of the time
    C. a milky discharge may be due to a pituitary adenoma
    D. benign duct papillomas are the most common cause of bloody discharges
    E. excision of the involved duct may be necessary to determine the etiology

12. The MOST frequent site for breast cancer to develop is the
    A. upper inner quadrant
    B. lower inner quadrant
    C. lower outer quadrant
    D. upper outer quadrant
    E. subareolar zone

13. The primary hormone responsible for lactogenesis is
   A. oxytocin
   B. estrogen
   C. prolactin
   D. luteinizing hormone (LH)
   E. follicle-stimulating hormone (FSH)

14. Diarrhea can be associated with all of the following EXCEPT
   A. Zollinger–Ellison syndrome
   B. hyperthyroidism
   C. carcinoid syndrome
   D. hyperparathyroidism
   E. medullary thyroid cancer

15. In which of the following categories of hyperaldosteronism is surgical treatment MOST likely to be successful?
   A. adrenocortical hyperplasia
   B. adrenocortical carcinoma
   C. adrenocortical adenoma
   D. glucocorticoid-suppressible hyperaldosteronism
   E. hyperaldosteronism unresponsive to spironolactone therapy

16. Which of the following is an INDIRECT action of parathyroid hormone?
   A. stimulation of osteoclastic bone resorption
   B. retardation of renal tubular reabsorption of phosphorus, resulting in phosphaturia
   C. enhanced gastrointestinal absorption of calcium
   D. a decrease in calcium clearance in the kidney
   E. stimulation of hydroxylation of 25-hydroxyvitamin D

17. The median survival of untreated patients with breast cancer is
   A. 8 months
   B. 1 1/2 years
   C. 2 1/2 years
   D. 5 years
   E. not known

18. The risk of bilateral breast cancer is HIGHEST if the first breast shows
  A. inflammatory carcinoma
  B. lobular carcinoma
  C. medullary carcinoma
  D. infiltrating ductal carcinoma
  E. Paget's disease

19. All of the following are true statements concerning Paget's disease of the nipple EXCEPT
  A. it is very uncommon, accounting for only 2% of all breast cancers
  B. it is an in situ squamous cell malignancy of the nipple
  C. it is an eczematoid lesion
  D. it has a better prognosis than the majority of other breast cancers
  E. it can be confused with malignant melanoma histologically

20. When stage I breast cancer is treated by partial mastectomy and axillary dissection, further therapy should include
  A. nothing
  B. chemotherapy
  C. antiestrogen agents
  D. radiation of the affected breast
  E. oophorectomy if premenopausal

21. Which of the following statements about milk lines is FALSE?
  A. they are common to all mammals
  B. between 2% and 6% of human females have an accessory nipple or extramammary breast tissue
  C. milk lines are derived from endoderm
  D. they extend from the axilla to the inguinal region
  E. none of the above

22. A 38-year-old patient presents with a unilateral 1-cm thyroid nodule. She is clinically euthyroid and has no family history of thyroid pathology. Physical exam fails to uncover any lymphadenopathy or associated tenderness. Possible next steps in your approach to this patient's care may include all of the following EXCEPT
    A. technetium thyroid scan
    B. needle aspiration
    C. ultrasonography
    D. suppression of the nodule with oral L-thyroxine
    E. obtain serum for determination of T_4 level

23. All of the following statements concerning prolactinomas are true EXCEPT
    A. they are the most frequently occurring posterior pituitary tumors
    B. they present clinically most commonly in females
    C. their most common presentation is secondary amenorrhea
    D. they can cause chiasmal compression and visual compromise
    E. they can be successfully treated with bromocriptine

24. The syndrome of multiple endocrine neoplasia (MEN) type II is an association of all of the following EXCEPT
    A. multiple neuromas
    B. pituitary tumors
    C. pheochromocytomas
    D. medullary carcinoma of the thyroid
    E. parathyroid hyperplasia

25. A 42-year-old patient presents to the emergency room with intractable nausea and vomiting, oliguria, muscle weakness, and drowsiness. Laboratory values reveal a BUN of 42, creatinine of 2.1, and a calcium of 15.3 mg/dL. Appropriate initial management would be
    A. hemodialysis
    B. fluid restriction and furosemide
    C. intravenous saline and furosemide
    D. intravenous phosphate
    E. mithramycin

26. Gynecomastia is associated with which of the following conditions?
    A. diazepam usage
    B. puberty
    C. aging
    D. cirrhosis
    E. all of the above

27. The 62-year-old patient who has the screening mammogram shown in Figure 4.1 should
    A. undergo immediate mastectomy
    B. undergo a biopsy of only palpable abnormalities
    C. return for a repeat mammogram in one year
    D. undergo a mammographically directed breast biopsy
    E. have an ultrasound exam of the suspicious area

Figure 4.1

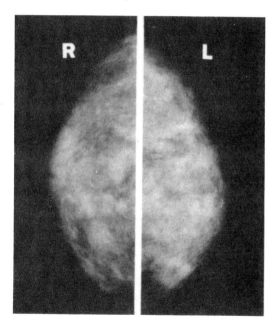

28. Which of the following studies is most effective in differentiating between solid and cystic lesions?
    A. screening mammography
    B. xeromammography
    C. ultrasonography
    D. thermography
    E. none of the above

29. All of the following statements concerning response of the breast to the hormonal changes associated with pregnancy are true EXCEPT
    A. ducts and lobules proliferate under the influence of increased estrogen and progesterone
    B. increased oxytocin levels induce the synthesis of milk fats during the last trimester
    C. the alveoli are filled with colloid during the second trimester
    D. connective and adipose tissue is replaced by proliferating glandular epithelium
    E. the alveoli are filled with colostrum in the third trimester

30. The MOST common type of congenital adrenal hyperplasia is due to
    A. deficiency of 11-hydroxylase
    B. deficiency of 17-hydroxylase
    C. deficiency of 21-hydroxylase
    D. excessive secretion of adrenocorticotropic hormone (ACTH)
    E. adrenal virilizing tumors

31. All of the following are true about papillary carcinoma of the thyroid EXCEPT
    A. it is the slowest growing malignant tumor of the thyroid
    B. it may change into the anaplastic variety
    C. it metastasizes primarily by hematogenous spread
    D. it is dependent on thyroid-stimulating hormone (TSH) stimulation
    E. it has a tendency to become more malignant with age

32. A 31-year-old G_1P_1 female presents with a unilateral serosanguinous nipple discharge. She has no palpable abnormalities on physical exam. The most likely diagnosis is
   A. ductal carcinoma in situ
   B. fibroadenoma
   C. cystosarcoma phyllodes
   D. intraductal papilloma
   E. medullary carcinoma

33. All of the following statements are true concerning the physiologic properties of parathyroid hormone EXCEPT
   A. it increases the reabsorption of calcium in the kidney
   B. it exerts its cellular effects via stimulation of adenylate cyclase
   C. its biologic activity is found within the first 34 N-terminal amino acid residues
   D. its secretion is regulated in part by the pituitary gland
   E. it decreases the reabsorption of phosphorus in the kidney

34. All of the following statements are true concerning thyroid storm EXCEPT
   A. it may be precipitated by trauma, infection, or acidosis
   B. it may be treated with large doses of intravenous sodium or potassium iodide
   C. cortisol is useful in therapy
   D. intravenous dantrolene is used to control the associated hyperthermia
   E. propranolol is useful for antagonizing the sympathetic effects

35. A 46-year-old male presents with recurrent episodes of severe headaches and sweating. Physical examination reveals a blood pressure of 170/95, a pulse of 95, and a thyroid nodule. Which of the following laboratory results would you expect to be elevated?
   A. thyroid-stimulating hormone
   B. urinary 5-hydroxyindoleacetic acid
   C. plasma serotonin
   D. urinary catecholamines
   E. serum thyroxine level

36. All of the following statements concerning the Zollinger–Ellison syndrome are true EXCEPT

   A. it can be a component of the MEN type I syndrome
   B. H$_2$-receptor antagonists are successful in the long-term management of acid hypersecretion
   C. the gastrin-secreting tumors rarely metastasize
   D. the ratio of basal acid output to maximal acid output is high compared with normal patients
   E. serum gastrin levels rise significantly in response to injected secretin or calcium

37. A 45-year-old patient presents with a tender breast mass of ten days' duration. Her family history is negative for breast cancer. Her last menstrual period ended 3 1/2 weeks ago, and today's mammogram exhibits no signs of malignancy. All of the following are appropriate management options EXCEPT

   A. reexamine her in 10 days
   B. reassure her that this is just a premenstrual change and resume routine screening
   C. obtain an ultrasound exam of the nodule
   D. schedule her for an excisional biopsy
   E. perform needle aspiration

38. A 42-year-old female presents with fatigue, weight gain, hirsutism, and acne. Physical examination reveals an elevated blood pressure, slender arms and legs with multiple bruises, and a "puffy" face. The most useful endocrine screening test for evaluation of this patient would be

   A. plasma ACTH
   B. high-dose dexamethasone suppression test
   C. 24-hour urine collection for free cortisol
   D. plasma cortisol
   E. plasma aldosterone

39. A 42-year-old man experiences multiple episodes of confusion, disorientation, and incoherence, usually occurring prior to mealtime. After eating, his erratic behavior totally resolves. He has no history of alcohol abuse and takes no medications. All of the following statements concerning his condition are true EXCEPT

   A. his fasting serum insulin:glucose ratio is elevated
   B. he most likely has a solitary benign tumor

C. a glucagon-secreting islet cell tumor is the cause of his reactive hypoglycemia

D. his fasting blood glucose is probably less than 50 mg/100 mL

E. he may require a surgical resection

40. Which of the following conditions LEAST warrants a breast biopsy for diagnosis?
A. an inverted nipple
B. bilateral green-colored nipple discharge
C. eczematous changes of the nipple
D. a nonpalpable mammographic abnormality
E. spontaneous unilateral single-duct nipple discharge

DIRECTIONS (Questions 41 through 69): The group of questions below consists of lettered headings followed by a list of numbered words, phrases, or statements. For each numbered word, phrase, or statement, select the ONE lettered heading that is most closely associated with it. Each lettered heading may be used once, more than once, or not at all.

Questions 41 through 43

A. cortisol
B. androgens
C. aldosterone
D. progesterone
E. epinephrine

41. Zona glomerulosa

42. Adrenal medulla

43. Zona fasciculata

Questions 44 and 45

    A. gastrinoma
    B. insulinoma
    C. VIPoma
    D. glucagonoma
    E. somatostatinoma

44. Beta-cell tumor of the pancreas

45. Alpha-cell tumor of the pancreas

Questions 46 and 47

    A. cystosarcoma phyllodes
    B. Paget's disease
    C. mild epithelial hyperplasia
    D. lobular carcinoma in-situ
    E. Mondor's disease

46. Considered a "marker" of increased risk for the development of subsequent invasive carcinoma

47. Usually presents as a large tumor

Questions 48 through 50

    A. psammoma bodies
    B. rapidly fatal once diagnosed
    C. calcitonin
    D. metastasizes primarily by hematogenous spread
    E. occurs primarily in elderly patients

48. Follicular carcinoma of the thyroid

49. Papillary carcinoma of the thyroid

50. Medullary carcinoma of the thyroid

Questions 51 through 53

    A. suppressed ACTH production
    B. normal ACTH production
    C. excessive pituitary ACTH production
    D. ectopic ACTH production
    E. none of the above

51. Oat cell carcinoma

52. Cushing's disease

53. Iatrogenic hypercortisolism

Questions 54 and 55

    A. $T_1N_0M_0$
    B. $T_1N_1M_0$
    C. $T_2N_0M_0$
    D. $T_2N_1M_0$
    E. none of the above

54. Describes a 2.5-cm breast cancer with no evidence of regional or distant metastases

55. Describes a breast cancer which presented with a 1-cm skin ulceration

Questions 56 through 59
    A. liothyronine
    B. propranolol
    C. propylthiouracil
    D. radioactive iodine
    E. subtotal thyroidectomy

56. Risk of agranulocytosis

57. Highest recurrence rate of hyperthyroidism

58. Highest potential risk of hypoparathyroidism

59. Highest potential risk of hypothyroidism

Questions 60 through 62
    A. clonidine
    B. levophed
    C. phenoxybenzamine
    D. phentolamine
    E. propanolol

60. Should not be given to patients with pheochromocytomas until after alpha blockade is established

61. Alpha-adrenergic blocking agent used to prepare patients with pheochromocytomas for surgery

62. Intravenous alpha blocking agent used intraoperatively during pheochromocytoma resections

Questions 63 through 69
The questions in this section refer to lettered choices contained in Figure 4.2.

63. Hypercalcemia of malignancy

64. Primary hyperparathyroidism

65. Pseudohypoparathyroidism

66. Hypoparathyroidism

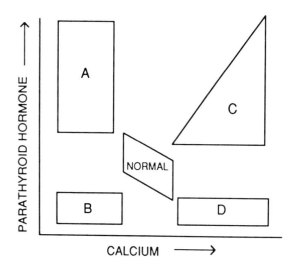

67. Sarcoidosis

68. Secondary hyperparathyroidism

69. Vitamin A intoxication

Breast and Endocrine Surgery

Answers and Comments

1. (D) Infertile women and women who delay their first pregnancy until after age 30 have an increased incidence of breast cancer. An early pregnancy and/or early castration diminishes this risk, which is believed to be related to prolonged exposure to estrogen. Fried, high-fat foods can almost double the risk of developing breast cancer. (**Ref. 1,** p. 517; **Ref. 2,** pp. 553–555; **Ref. 6,** p. 294)

2. (B) Infiltrating ductal carcinoma accounts for 75% to 80% of all breast cancer. (**Ref. 1,** p. 526; **Ref. 2,** p. 563)

3. (D) The synthesis, storage, and release of thyroid hormone occurs in the follicular cells. Iodide is trapped from serum and oxidized to iodine. It is then incorporated into tyrosine (organification) to form either monoiodotyrosine or diiodotyrosine; these two couple to form T_3 or T_4, which are then released after hydrolysis in colloid into the circulation. (**Ref. 1,** pp. 560–561; **Ref. 2,** pp. 1616–1617)

4. (B) Papillary carcinoma (pure and papillary–follicular mixed) accounts for 60% to 70% of all thyroid cancers. (**Ref. 2,** p. 1633; **Ref. 6,** p. 281)

5. **(B)** Prior surgery on the neck, especially thyroid surgery, accounts for the greater majority of hypoparathyroidism in adults. Injury to or removal of the parathyroid glands is the etiology. (**Ref. 1,** p. 613; **Ref. 2,** p. 1673)

6. **(D)** Although the factors that control insulin secretion from the beta cells in the islets of Langerhans are multiple, the most important is an elevation of the extracellular blood glucose. (**Ref. 1,** p. 1079; **Ref. 2,** p. 1405)

7. **(D)** Cholesterol is the basic precursor of all the adrenal steroids, and through a series of hydroxylations, dehydrogenations, and isomerization reactions, is transformed into progesterone, testosterone, cortisol, and aldosterone. (**Ref. 1,** pp. 627–628; **Ref. 2,** p. 1564)

8. **(B)** Oxytocin and vasopressin are synthesized in the hypothalamus and migrate down the neurohypophyseal tract to the posterior pituitary. (**Ref. 1,** p. 618; **Ref. 2,** pp. 1549–1550)

9. **(A)** Mammographic evidence of malignancy includes fine punctate calcification in a localized area, thickened overlying skin, and local asymmetric increased tissue density. Large coarse calcifications are usually associated with benign lesions. (**Ref. 1,** pp. 519–520; **Ref. 2,** pp. 540–544; **Ref. 6,** p. 296)

10. **(D)** Acute mastitis occurs frequently during lactation, with infection resulting from staphylococci or streptococci entering the breast through abraded or lacerated nipple surfaces. (**Ref. 1,** p. 523; **Ref. 2,** pp. 545–546)

11. **(B)** Benign duct papillomas account for the majority of bloody nipple discharges, while malignancy is the cause in only 10% to 30%. Prolactinomas can cause galactorrhea. (**Ref. 1,** pp. 515–516; **Ref. 2,** pp. 540, 551–552)

12. **(D)** Forty percent to fifty percent of breast cancers develop in the upper outer quadrant, due to the relatively larger volume of breast tissue in this location. Centrally located cancers account for 15% to 20% of cases. (**Ref. 2,** p. 562; **Ref. 6,** p. 297)

13. (C) Following parturition, the fall in estrogen and progesterone levels allow prolactin to stimulate the production of milk. Oxytocin initiates contraction of the smooth muscle cells surrounding the breast alveoli, compressing them and causing expulsion of the milk. (**Ref. 1,** p. 515; **Ref. 2,** pp. 537–538)

14. (D) Patients with Zollinger–Ellison syndrome experience diarrhea due to increased serum gastrin levels, while carcinoid tumors secrete serotonin which causes hypermotility. Hypermotility and diarrhea can be seen in some thyrotoxic patients, and secretory diarrhea is occasionally associated with medullary cancer, which secretes prostaglandin. Constipation, not diarrhea, is more likely to be associated with hyperparathyroidism. (**Ref. 1,** pp. 569, 602, 870, 1100; **Ref. 2,** pp. 1176, 1428, 1620, 1649)

15. (C) In patients with hyperaldosteronism secondary to a benign adenoma, surgical resection is curative 60% to 90% of the time. Idiopathic hyperplasia is best treated medically; patients who fail spironolactone therapy require subtotal or total adrenalectomies and usually respond poorly. Adrenocortical carcinoma is treated surgically, but the long-term survival is dismal. (**Ref. 1,** pp. 634–636; **Ref. 2,** p. 1581)

16. (C) Parathyroid hormone increases serum calcium by releasing it from bone, by increasing calcium reabsorption and phosphate clearance in the kidney, and by stimulating conversion of 25-hydroxyvitamin D to 1,25-dihydroxyvitamin D. The latter is responsible for the enhancement of gastrointestinal absorption of calcium from the diet. (**Ref. 1,** p. 600; **Ref. 2,** pp. 1646–1648)

17. (C) The median survival of untreated breast cancer is between two and three years. (**Ref. 1,** p. 528; **Ref. 2,** p. 554)

18. (B) Lobular carcinoma of the breast is associated with a higher incidence of either invasive or in situ lesions in the opposite breast as often as 20% of the time. (**Ref. 1,** p. 526; **Ref. 6,** p. 302)

19. (B) Paget's disease of the nipple is an uncommon presentation of an underlying intraductal or invasive ductal breast carcinoma. It appears as a chronic, eczematoid eruption and generally has a somewhat better prognosis than the majority of lesions because the visible changes of the nipple promote early consultation and diagnosis. Microscopically, this lesion can be confused with pagetoid intraepithelial malignant melanoma, and occasionally immunohistochemistry must be employed to demonstrate carcinoembryonic antigen (CEA) within the breast cancer cells. (**Ref. 2,** pp. 562–563; **Ref. 3,** pp. 311–312)

20. **(D)**   When breast cancer is treated by partial mastectomy, the remaining breast tissue on the affected side will develop recurrent disease 24% to 36% of the time unless treated with radiation therapy. This is due to the multicentric nature of breast cancer. Any additional adjuvant therapy will be determined based on the patient's age, menopausal status, and the histological parameters of her tumor. (**Ref. 1,** pp. 530–533; **Ref. 2,** p. 578)

21. **(C)**   The milk lines, or mammary ridges, are two bands of thickened ectoderm from which breast tissue ultimately develops over the pectoral muscles. Failure of the remaining milk lines to regress prior to birth results in the appearance of accessory nipples and/or extramammary breast tissue. (**Ref. 1,** p. 511; **Ref. 2,** pp. 531–532)

22. **(D)**   Although the majority of solitary thyroid nodules are benign, it is important to establish cytologic or histologic proof of benignity. Many thyroid cancers have TSH receptor sites and will regress slightly in size with L-thyroxine suppression therapy. Further characterization of this patient's nodule is indicated. (**Ref. 1,** pp. 582–584; **Ref. 2,** pp. 1630–1633)

23. **(A)**   Prolactinomas are anterior pituitary tumors. In females, cessation of menstrual periods occurs as the presenting symptom most frequently; only 50% of amenorrheic patients have associated galactorrhea. Large tumors compress the optic chiasm and cause visual field reductions. Tumors can be treated surgically, medically with bromocriptine, or with radiotherapy. (**Ref. 1,** pp. 620, 623–624; **Ref. 2,** pp. 1553–1554)

24. **(B)**   Type II MEN syndrome is an association of medullary thyroid carcinoma with pheochromocytomas. Type IIa includes parathyroid hyperplasia, and type IIb is associated with multiple mucosal neuromas. (**Ref. 1,** p. 592; **Ref. 2,** p. 325)

25. **(C)** Acute hypercalcemic crisis can be caused by hyperparathyroidism (benign or malignant), or assorted malignancies. Therapy consists of fluid rehydration with saline followed by furosemide to promote renal excretion of calcium. Intravenous phosphate can cause calcium precipitation in the lungs; mithramycin's calcium-lowering effects take 24 hours to occur. **(Ref. 1,** pp. 606–607; **Ref. 2,** pp. 1649–1650)

26. **(E)** Gynecomastia can be a normal physiologic change seen at birth, puberty, and senescence. During all three of these periods, there is a relative excess of estrogens in relation to circulating testosterone. Certain disease states, such as cirrhosis and endocrine disorders, can also initiate a relative estrogen excess. Drugs that inhibit the synthesis or action of testosterone may result in gynecomastia. These include cimetidine, phenytoin, spironolactone, and diazepam. **(Ref. 1,** p. 515; **Ref. 2,** p. 539; **Ref. 3,** p. 301)

27. **(D)** The punctate microcalcifications that are seen in the left breast are associated with malignancy 20% of the time. Since this is usually not a palpable lesion, mammographic localization must be done to guide the surgeon to the suspicious area. **(Ref. 1,** pp. 519–520; **Ref. 2,** pp. 541, 545, 568)

28. **(C)** Although the resolution of ultrasonography is inferior to that of mammography and xeromammography, it is capable of distinguishing cystic from solid lesions. Thermography detects transmitted heat from vascular carcinomas, but due to its low specificity is no longer utilized. **(Ref. 2,** p. 544; **Ref. 6,** p. 296)

29. **(B)** Prolactin stimulates limited synthesis of milk fats and proteins during late pregnancy (lactogenesis). The presence of cortisol, insulin, and growth hormone are required for this action. Oxytocin causes smooth muscle contraction necessary for the ejection of milk (lactation). **(Ref. 1,** p. 515; **Ref. 2,** pp. 537–538)

30. **(C)** Deficiency of 21-hydroxylase is the most common cause of congenital adrenal hyperplasia. Partial deficiency results in a simple virilizing form of adrenal hyperplasia, and a complete deficiency causes a salt-losing variety which can be life-threatening. **(Ref. 1,** p. 636; **Ref. 2,** p. 1582)

31. **(C)** Papillary carcinoma metastasizes primarily to the lymph nodes in the neck; only 4% to 20% of patients will ultimately develop metastases in lung, bone, or other soft tissues. In the elderly, papillary cancer is more virulent, and it is often closely associated with the development of anaplastic thyroid cancer in these patients. (**Ref. 2,** pp. 1633–1635, 1639–1640)

32. **(D)** Intraductal papillomas are the etiology for the majority of cancer presenting with serosanguinous nipple discharge. However, since cancers can account for 10% to 30% of blood-stained nipple discharge, biopsy is warranted. (**Ref. 1,** pp. 515–516; **Ref. 2,** pp. 551–552)

33. **(D)** The secretion of parathyroid hormone is regulated by the circulating concentration of calcium. There is no pituitary hormone that either stimulates or inhibits its secretion. (**Ref. 1,** p. 600; **Ref. 2,** pp. 1647–1648)

34. **(D)** Thyroid storm, although a rare event, carries a 10% mortality. The fever that is part of thyrotoxic crisis is treated with a cooling blanket and acetaminophen; dantrolene is not used. The other treatment modalities listed are also vital. (**Ref. 1,** p. 573; **Ref. 2,** p. 1643)

35. **(D)** Patients with pheochromocytomas can present with either paroxysmal or sustained hypertension, headaches, and sweating; a 24-hour urine collection for catecholamines and their metabolites will aid in making the diagnosis. A toxic thyroid adenoma would be rare in a male and does not cause hypertension or headaches. His thyroid nodule may be a medullary cancer. (**Ref. 1,** pp. 569, 642, 871; **Ref. 2,** pp. 1589–1590)

36. **(C)** Since the acid hypersecretion in Zollinger–Ellison patients can usually be controlled medically, most of these patients die from metastatic disease unless a curative resection can be achieved early in the course. The ratio of basal acid output (BAO) to maximum acid output (MAO) is in excess of 0.6. (**Ref. 1,** pp. 1099–1102; **Ref. 2,** pp. 1427–1428; **Ref. 4,** p. 255)

37. **(B)** At a minimum, she should return at the conclusion of her next menstrual period (5 to 10 days) for a repeat exam. Although

it is possible that this new lesion represents premenstrual nodularity, this should not be assumed without further proof. Either total disappearance of the nodule, confirmation of its cystic nature, or histologic determination of benign nature is required. (**Ref. 1,** p. 515; **Ref. 2,** pp. 537, 544, 568)

38. **(C)**   The most reliable initial test to screen for Cushing's syndrome is a 24-hour urinary free cortisol determination. Plasma cortisol levels vary significantly throughout the day (diurnal fluctuation), and it is sometimes possible to obtain a normal level in patients with hypercortisolism. (**Ref. 1,** p. 630; **Ref. 2,** p. 1571; **Ref. 4,** p. 269)

39. **(C)**   Insulinomas are beta islet cell tumors which are solitary and benign 80% of the time. Fasting hypoglycemia and an insulin:glucose ratio exceeding 0.3 are diagnostic. Surgery is the treatment of choice. Glucagonomas present with mild diabetes, not hypoglycemia, as part of their syndrome. (**Ref. 1,** pp. 1099, 1102–1103; **Ref. 2,** pp. 1426–1429; **Ref. 4,** p. 255)

40. **(B)**   Bilateral nonbloody nipple discharge is commonly associated with diffuse fibrocystic changes within the breasts. Unilateral single duct discharge heralds a more localized pathology, and a biopsy is necessary to differentiate a benign ductal papilloma from a carcinoma. An inverted nipple is often associated with a breast cancer, and Paget's disease is a relatively early indicator of an underlying malignancy as well. Any suspicious mammographic finding requires investigation, regardless of the lack of a mass on physical exam. (**Ref. 2,** pp. 545, 551, 562–566; **Ref. 4,** p. 261)

41. **(C)**   Aldosterone, a mineralocorticoid, is secreted in the zona glomerulosa and influences electrolyte balance. (**Ref. 2,** p. 1567; **Ref. 4,** p. 269)

42. **(E)**   Both epinephrine and norepinephrine are synthesized in the adrenal medulla. (**Ref. 2,** p. 1583; **Ref. 4,** p. 269)

43. **(A)**   The glucocorticoids, secreted in the zona fasciculata, are involved with protein and carbohydrate metabolism. (**Ref. 4,** p. 269)

44. **(B)**   Produces hypoglycemia if the insulin product is biologically active. The tumor is benign and solitary 80% of the time. (**Ref. 1,** p. 1099; **Ref. 2,** pp. 1426–1427; **Ref. 4,** p. 255)

45. **(D)**   A glucagonoma produces a syndrome of stomatitis, dermatitis, and mild diabetes mellitus. This tumor is usually malignant. (**Ref. 1,** pp. 1102–1103; **Ref. 2,** p. 1429

46. **(D)**   Women diagnosed with lobular carcinoma in situ are usually up to 15 years younger than those developing invasive breast cancer, and between 10% and 37% of women with LCIS will subsequently develop an invasive breast carcinoma more than 15 years later. Mild epithelial hyperplasia without atypia carries no increased risk for subsequent breast cancer. Mondor's disease is a thrombophlebitis of the superficial veins of the anterior chest wall and breast and is not associated with malignancy. (**Ref. 1,** pp. 526, 536–537; **Ref. 2,** pp. 548–549, 560–561)

47. **(A)**   Cystosarcoma phyllodes, or phyllodes tumors, present as large circumscribed masses measuring 4 to 10 cm in diameter. Histologically, they resemble fibroadenomas and exhibit benign behavior 80% to 90% of the time. (**Ref. 1,** p. 544; **Ref. 2,** p. 551; **Ref. 4,** p. 261)

48. **(D)**   Only 10% to 15% of patients with follicular cancer of the thyroid develop lymph node metastases; the most common sites of metastases are lung and bone. Both papillary and medullary cancers spread primarily to lymph nodes. (**Ref. 1,** p. 587; **Ref. 2,** p. 1636)

49. **(A)**   Papillary thyroid cancers may contain characteristic localized deposits of calcium arranged in concentric layers called psammoma bodies. (**Ref. 2,** p. 1634)

50. **(C)**   Medullary thyroid cancer arises from calcitonin-producing parafollicular cells. (**Ref. 1,** p. 592; **Ref. 2,** pp. 1638–1639; **Ref. 4,** p. 283)

51. **(D)**   Cushing's syndrome (hypercortisolism) can result from the ectopic production of ACTH from nonadrenal tumors, such as oat cell carcinoma of the lung, carcinoid tumors in the bronchi, and

medullary thyroid cancer. (**Ref. 1,** pp. 630–632; **Ref. 2,** p. 1569; **Ref. 4,** p. 269)

52. (**C**)   Cushing's disease is hypercortisolism due to the excessive production of ACTH by a pituitary neoplasm. (**Ref. 1,** p. 632; **Ref. 2,** p. 1569; **Ref. 4,** p. 269)

53. (**A**)   The most common cause of Cushing's syndrome is chronic administration of synthetic corticosteroids. This suppresses the pituitary production of ACTH. (**Ref. 1,** p. 630; **Ref. 2,** pp. 1568–1569)

54. (**C**) $T_2N_0M_0$ describes a stage II, node-negative breast cancer measuring more than 2 cm but less than 5 cm in diameter. (**Ref. 1,** pp. 527–529; **Ref. 2,** pp. 557–559; **Ref. 4,** pp. 263–264)

55. (**E**)   Any breast cancer, regardless of size, which presents with fixation to the chest wall, peau d'orange (edematous skin changes) or ulceration of the skin is classified as T_4, signifying a locally advanced malignancy. (**Ref. 1,** pp. 527–529; **Ref. 2,** pp. 557–559; **Ref. 4,** pp. 263–264)

56. (**C**)   Drug rash, fever, and agranulocytosis are potential reactions to propylthiouracil and methimazole. (**Ref. 1,** p. 570; **Ref. 2,** pp. 1621–1622)

57. (**C**)   Propylthiouracil (and methimazole) cause permanent remission of hyperthyroidism in only a minority of patients (less than 40%). Antithyroid drugs are used mainly to render patients euthyroid prior to instituting ablative therapy. Propranolol is added if tachycardia is persistent. (**Ref. 1,** p. 570; **Ref. 2,** pp. 1621–1622; **Ref. 4,** p. 281)

58. (**E**)   Subtotal thyroidectomy carries a small but real risk of hypoparathyroidism due to injury to the glands. Radioactive iodine and antithyroid drugs do not have a noticeable effect on the parathyroid glands. (**Ref. 1,** p. 571; **Ref. 2,** p. 1622)

59. (**D**)   When treating hyperthyroidism with radioiodine, the long-term risk of hypothyroidism is 40% to 70%, compared to only 20% for surgery. (**Ref. 1,** pp. 570–571; **Ref. 2,** p. 1622; **Ref. 4,** p. 281)

60. **(E)** Beta-blocking agents are indicated to treat tachycardia, arrhythmias, and high epinephrine levels in patients with pheochromocytomas; starting them prior to the establishment of adequate alpha-blockade could result in life-threatening hypertensive crises. (**Ref. 1,** pp. 645–646; **Ref. 2,** pp. 1591–1592)

61. **(C)** Phenoxybenzamine, and more recently prazosin, are oral alpha-blocking agents used to stabilize pheochromocytoma patients preoperatively. (**Ref. 1,** pp. 645–646; **Ref. 2,** p. 1592; **Ref. 4,** p. 273)

62. **(D)** Phentolamine is an alpha-blocking agent used intravenously by anesthesiologists to control hypertensive episodes during pheochromocytoma resections. Nitroprusside is another shorter-acting drug that can be used for this purpose as well. Levophed is used if needed to reverse sudden hypotension intraoperatively in these patients. (**Ref. 1,** p. 646; **Ref. 2,** p. 1592; **Ref. 4,** p. 273)

63. **(D)** Elevated calcium levels due to bony metastases or certain nonendocrine tumors suppress serum parathyroid hormone levels. (**Ref. 2,** pp. 1651–1652)

64. **(C)** Increased production of parathyroid hormone by adenomatous or hyperplastic glands elevates the serum calcium. (**Ref. 2,** p. 1650)

65. **(A)** These patients have defective parathyroid hormone receptors, so that the end organs are unresponsive to the parathyroid hormone (PTH). The end result is an elevated PTH level and hypocalcemia. (**Ref. 2,** p. 1674)

66. **(B)** Absent or hypofunctioning parathyroid glands. The most common cause is injury during neck surgery. (**Ref. 2,** p. 1673)

67. **(D)** Sarcoidosis and other granulomatous diseases produce a hydroxylase that converts vitamin D to an active metabolite, producing hypercalcemia. (**Ref. 4,** p. 285)

68. **(A)** Increased PTH secretion in secondary hyperparathyroidism is in response to a chronically low serum calcium brought about

by renal disease or malabsorption syndromes. (**Ref. 1,** p. 607; **Ref. 2,** p. 1658; **Ref. 4,** p. 287)

69. **(D)** Toxic levels of both vitamins A and D can cause hypercalcemia, which will suppress parathyroid hormone levels. (**Ref. 1,** p. 607; **Ref. 2,** p. 1652)

5

Urologic Surgery and Transplantation

Stephen H. Weinstein
Michael S. Callister

DIRECTIONS (Questions 1 through 45): Each of the questions or incomplete statements below is followed by five suggested answers or completions. Select the ONE that is best in each case.

Questions 1 through 9

1. On arrival at the hospital, a 38-year-old male victim of an automobile accident complains of abdominal pain. Physical exam reveals pain above the symphysis pubis, pelvic instability, and no blood at the urethral meatus. The best test for diagnosis of bladder rupture is
   A. cystoscopy
   B. intravenous pyelogram (IVP)
   C. cystogram
   D. failure of return of a measured quantity of fluid instilled
   E. blood in the urine

2. Ureteral injuries are LEAST common as a result of
   A. radical hysterectomy
   B. penetrating or blunt trauma
   C. abdominoperineal resection
   D. ureteroscopy
   E. radiation therapy of carcinoma of the cervix

3. A 20-year-old female complained of right flank pain. The IVP is
   shown in Figure 5.1. The diagnosis is
   A. bladder diverticulum
   B. ureterocele
   C. stone in ureterovesical junction
   D. tumor in ureter
   E. tumor in bladder

Figure 5.1

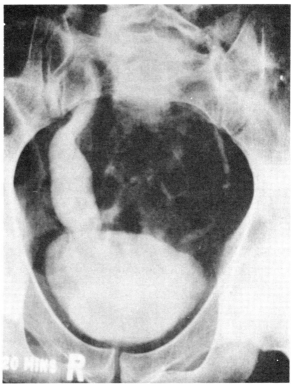

4. A couple seeks medical advice regarding their newborn son because they cannot feel testes in the scrotum. Regarding cryptorchidism as a cause for the empty scrotum, all of the following statements are correct EXCEPT

  A. it is often associated with inguinal hernia
  B. it is associated with torsion of the spermatic cord
  C. it is associated with tumor of the testes
  D. spontaneous descent of testes can occur
  E. surgical correction should be performed before age 2

5. Torsion of the spermatic cord

  A. occurs in young individuals
  B. is a benign condition, usually resolving spontaneously
  C. may be caused by epididymitis
  D. is often bilateral
  E. is associated with hematuria

6. A 65 year-old male with microscopic hematuria undergoes cystoscopy. Three 5-mm papillary lesions are found at the base of the bladder, and pathology of the biopsy returns as transitional cell carcinoma. These tumors are usually treated by

  A. transurethral resection
  B. segmental cystectomy
  C. total cystectomy
  D. radiotherapy
  E. suprapubic cystostomy and fulguration

7. During workup for microhematuria, an IVP shows aberrant renal pelvic architecture. Subsequent computed tomography (CT) scan reveals a 4-cm intraparenchymal mass that enhances with contrast and is consistent with carcinoma. The statement BEST characterizing renal cell carcinoma is

  A. it is more common in men
  B. it usually does not have a capsule
  C. it metastasizes predominantly by the lymphatic route
  D. it may cause fever due to secondary infection
  E. it is often bilateral

8. The statement that BEST characterizes cancer of the penis is
   A. it commonly metastasizes by the deep pelvic veins
   B. it is rare in men circumcised during infancy
   C. it involves the foreskin but not the glans
   D. para-aortic lymph nodes are usually involved
   E. radiotherapy is the treatment of choice

9. The statement that BEST characterizes retroperitoneal fibrosis is
   A. it involves females predominantly
   B. it does not cause symptoms
   C. it tends to cause ureteral obstruction
   D. it involves only the lumbar area
   E. it is sharply encapsulated

Questions 10 and 11

A 45 year-old woman has recurrent renal calculi and has undergone multiple extracorporeal shock wave lithotripsy (ESWL) treatments.

10. Her stone disease may be related to all of the following EXCEPT
    A. vitamin D metabolism
    B. urea-splitting bacteria
    C. immobilization
    D. stenosis of ureteropelvic junction
    E. hyperthyroidism

11. This patient now comes to the emergency room with a history of acute onset of intense right flank pain. Urinalysis shows 10 to 20 RBCs per high power field, and subsequent IVP showed evidence of right ureteral obstruction with a 6-mm × 12-mm filling defect, but no evidence of calculi on the kidney, ureter, and bladder (KUB). Which of the following urinary calculi is radiolucent?
    A. calcium oxalate
    B. uric acid
    C. cystine stones
    D. triple phosphate stones (struvite)
    E. calcium phosphate

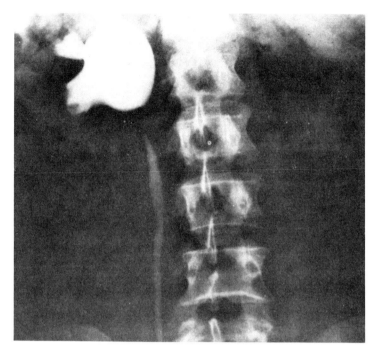

Figure 5.2

Questions 12 and 13

A 15 year-old male with a long history of intermittent right flank pain was admitted with a severe attack of pain, nausea, and vomiting. The IVP is shown in Figure 5.2.

12. The most common cause of the condition is
   A. aberrant renal artery
   B. calculus
   C. functional disorder of the ureteropelvic junction
   D. adhesions
   E. valves

13. Treatment of the condition shown in Figure 5.2 is
   A. nephrectomy
   B. nephropexy
   C. pyeloplasty
   D. partial nephrectomy
   E. internal drainage

Questions 14 through 25

14. Localized carcinoma of the prostate is BEST treated by which of the following modalities?
   A. bilateral orchiectomy
   B. estrogens
   C. orchiectomy followed by estrogens
   D. radical prostatectomy
   E. transurethral resection of the prostate

15. Infection with which of the following organisms commonly predisposes to urinary stone formation?
   A. *Escherichia coli*
   B. *Proteus vulgaris* and *Pseudomonas aeruginosa*
   C. *Streptococcus faecalis*
   D. *Mycobacterium tuberculosis*
   E. *Bacillus typhosus*

16. The MOST common manifestation of Wilms' tumor is
   A. abdominal mass
   B. loss of weight
   C. hematuria
   D. hypertension
   E. pathologic fracture of bone

17. The MOST common symptom of a renal parenchymal tumor in an adult is
   A. abdominal mass
   B. hematuria
   C. unexplained fever
   D. anemia
   E. hemoptysis due to metastases in the lung

18. Which of the following statements is correct with regard to the venous return from testes (spermatic veins)?
    A. the right and left veins join together and enter the vena cava
    B. the right one drains into the inferior vena cava and the left joins the left renal vein
    C. the right one joins the renal vein and the left joins the vena cava
    D. the vein on each side joins the renal vein on the same side
    E. the two veins join the inferior vena cava separately

19. A 75-year-old male arrives in the emergency room with a tender lower abdominal mass and inability to void urine during the preceding 12 hours. The MOST likely cause of his condition is
    A. carcinoma of the prostate
    B. chronic prostatitis
    C. benign hyperplasia of the prostate
    D. stricture of the urethra
    E. prostatic abscess

20. In differentiating a renal cyst from a renal tumor, which of the following radiologic studies is MOST definitive?
    A. CT scan
    B. retrograde pyelography
    C. intravenous pyelogram (IVP)
    D. renal scan
    E. renal ultrasound

21. During a periodic health evaluation, a 67 year-old male is noted to have microhematuria. An IVP and cystogram is performed. These tests show radiologic features of benign hypertrophy of the prostate (BPH), which might include all of the following EXCEPT
    A. filling defect at base of the bladder
    B. calcification of the prostate
    C. diverticula of the bladder
    D. bladder stones
    E. ureteric dilation

22. In benign prostatic hypertrophy, all of the following are indications for prostatectomy EXCEPT
    A. poor stream
    B. annoying frequency and nocturia
    C. large amount of infected residual urine
    D. enlarged prostate
    E. secondary diverticula or stone

23. Advantages of transurethral prostatectomy over open prostatectomy include all of the following EXCEPT
    A. lower mortality and morbidity
    B. bladder diverticula can be removed
    C. less risk of wound healing or urinary fistula
    D. shorter period of catheterization
    E. fewer bleeding problems

24. The transabdominal approach to the kidney is advisable in
    A. calculus disease
    B. tuberculosis
    C. tumor
    D. cystic disease
    E. hydronephrosis

25. The BEST test for diagnosis of chronic prostatitis is
    A. palpation only
    B. urine culture
    C. cystoscopy
    D. microscopic examination of prostatic secretions
    E. IVP

Questions 26 and 27

A 58 year-old male with a long history of cigarette smoking has transitional cell carcinoma of the bladder.

26. The MOST accurate technique for staging bladder tumors is
    A. IVP
    B. urine cytology
    C. transurethral biopsy

D. bimanual examination

E. cystogram

27. Since initial diagnosis, the patient has had multiple recurrent superficial tumors and carcinoma in situ. These bladder tumors may be treated with all of the following topical agents. Response rates are BEST with

A. bacille Calmette-Guérin (BCG)

B. thio-TEPA

C. cis-platinum

D. mitomycin-C

E. doxorubicin

Questions 28 through 45

28. In a patient with gross hematuria, a radiolucent filling defect in the renal pelvis on intravenous pyelogram may be due to

A. nonopaque calculus

B. blood clot

C. tumor

D. extrinsic compression

E. all of the above

29. High ligation of the internal spermatic vein(s) in the treatment of infertility is recommended for

A. Kallman's syndrome (hypogonadotrophic hypogonadism)

B. spermatogenic arrest

C. obstructive azospermia

D. chronic epididymitis

E. varicocele

30. Which of the following correlates LEAST well with significant bladder outlet obstruction secondary to benign prostatic hyperplasia?

A. bladder wall trabeculation on cystoscopy

B. size of the prostate on rectal examination

C. peak urinary flow rate

D. residual urine

E. recurrent infections

31. Hypospadias is generally associated with all of the following EX-CEPT
    A. dystopic urethral meatus
    B. hooded dorsal foreskin
    C. ventral curvature or chordee of the penile shaft
    D. upper urinary tract anomalies
    E. flattened glans

32. A 65-year-old male patient with coronary artery disease is being evaluated for sexual impotence. The patient's history reveals that he has been unable to achieve sufficient erection for vaginal penetration for approximately 2 years. He has a long history of cigarette smoking, and has moderate claudication after walking half a block. Which of the following would NOT be indicated as definitive treatment?
    A. vacuum erection device
    B. inflatable penile prosthesis
    C. psychological counseling
    D. penile injection therapy
    E. vascular reconstruction

33. A patient with gross hematuria comes in for evaluation. Your differential diagnosis generally includes all of the following clinical disorders EXCEPT
    A. cystitis in women
    B. calculus disease
    C. cancer of the prostate
    D. cancer of the kidney
    E. cancer of the bladder

34. In uncomplicated cystitis, the MOST common organism found on urine culture is
    A. group B streptococcus
    B. *Escherichia coli*
    C. *Klebsiella*
    D. *Staphylococcus aureus*
    E. chlamydia

35. A 50-year-old woman is being evaluated for right flank pain. She has a history of calcium oxalate renal calculi. An IVP shows a 1-cm, nonobstructing stone in the right renal pelvis. The treatment of choice is

   A. open surgical removal

   B. dissolution therapy

   C. percutaneous nephrostolithotomy

   D. extracorporeal shockwave lithotripsy (ESWL)

   E. ureteroscopic laser disintegration

36. Urodynamic studies to assess the neuromuscular function of the bladder and bladder outlet may include all of the following tests EXCEPT

   A. urethral pressure profile

   B. cystometrogram

   C. uroflowmetry

   D. dynamic cavernosometry

   E. sphincter electromyography

37. In a patient with ureteral obstruction secondary to radiation fibrosis requiring immediate decompression, which of the following is the procedure of choice when retrograde catheterization is not possible?

   A. ureteral reimplantation

   B. open nephrostomy

   C. nephrectomy

   D. cutaneous ureterostomy

   E. percutaneous nephrostomy

38. Which of the following studies is NOT generally indicated in the evaluation of a patient with significant blunt trauma and gross hematuria?

   A. retrograde cystography

   B. cystoscopy

   C. retrograde urethrography

   D. infusion pyelography

   E. CT scan

39. Which of the following provides the most accurate assessment of renal function?
   A. blood urea nitrogen (BUN)
   B. creatinine clearance
   C. IVP
   D. free water clearance
   E. concentrating ability

40. A 71-year-old female complains of recent onset pneumaturia. A CT scan is consistent with, but not diagnostic of, a vesicoenteric fistula. The MOST common cause of vesicoenteric fistulae is
   A. colorectal malignancy
   B. iatrogenic
   C. inflammatory bowel disease
   D. bladder malignancy
   E. sigmoid diverticulitis

41. Stress urinary incontinence in multiparous women may be successfully treated by all of the following EXCEPT
   A. vaginal urethral suspension
   B. anticholinergic medication
   C. Marshall–Marchetti urethral suspension
   D. sympathomimetic agents
   E. anterior urethropexy

42. In cadaveric renal transplantation in adults, all of the following surgical techniques are commonly employed EXCEPT
   A. intraperitoneal placement of the kidney
   B. end-to-end renal artery to recipient internal iliac artery anastomosis
   C. end-to-side renal vein to recipient external iliac vein anastomosis
   D. end-to-side renal artery to recipient external iliac artery anastomosis
   E. submucosal ureteral anastomosis to bladder

43. All of the following agents may be part of conventional immunosuppression in cadaver kidney recipients. Which one has been MOST responsible for improved graft survival statistics?
   A. antilymphocyte serum (ALS)
   B. cyclosporine

    C. prednisone
    D. azathioprine (Imuran)
    E. OKT-3

44. The following signs and symptoms are commonly seen with acute renal transplant rejection EXCEPT
    A. gross hematuria
    B. graft tenderness
    C. fever
    D. decreased urine sodium
    E. decreased renal function

45. Which of the following early or late complications of renal transplantation is seen with reasonable frequency in a busy transplant practice?
    A. lymphocele
    B. pneumocystis carinii infection
    C. renal transplant artery stenosis
    D. lymphoma and skin cancers
    E. all of the above

DIRECTIONS (Questions 46 through 58): Each group of questions below consists of lettered headings followed by a list of numbered words, phrases, or statements. For each numbered word, phrase, or statement, select the ONE lettered heading that is most closely associated with it. Each lettered heading may be selected once, more than once, or not at all.

Questions 46 through 49

    A. varicocele
    B. hydrocele
    C. spermatocele
    D. ureterocele
    E. urethral diverticulum

46. Cobra-head deformity

47. Usually on left side

48. Cyst of epididymis

49. Common in children

Questions 50 through 54

    A. embryonal carcinoma
    B. seminoma
    C. interstitial cell tumor (Leydig cell tumor)
    D. choriocarcinoma
    E. teratoma

50. Generally treated with radiation therapy

51. Precocious sexual maturation in boys

52. Most common testicular tumor in childhood

53. Extremely invasive with early metastasis

54. Least malignant testicular tumor

Questions 55 through 58

    A. interstitial cystitis
    B. posterior urethral valves
    C. congenital adrenal hyperplasia
    D. duplicated ureter
    E. torsion of appendix testis

55. Diagnosed by voiding cystourethrography

56. Metanephric duct

57. Dimethyl sulfoxide (DMSO) treatment

58. Salt-losing tendency

Urologic Surgery and Transplantation

Answers and Comments

1. **(C)** A cystogram not only demonstrates the extent of the vesical rupture but also gives an indication as to whether it is an extraperitoneal or intraperitoneal rupture. (**Ref. 1,** p. 1452)

2. **(B)** As the ureters are deeply placed and well protected in the retroperitoneum, penetrating or blunt trauma rarely causes ureteral injury. Unfortunately, iatrogenic ureteral injury is relatively common. (**Ref. 1,** p. 1446; **Ref. 3,** p. 1722)

3. **(B)** The lesion shown is a dilated ureter with a cobra-head deformity and is due to a ureterocele. A ureterocele is a congenital abnormality and is due to stenosis of the ureteric orifice in the bladder. It is covered by ureteral epithelium inside and bladder epithelium outside. (**Ref. 2,** pp. 1772–1774; **Ref. 3,** p. 1703)

4. **(B)** Because the testis remains intra-abdominal, torsion of the cord does not occur. The undescended testis is often associated with an abnormal processus vaginalis that leads to inguinal hernia. The risk of malignancy in an undescended testis is 20 times more than in the normally descended one. (**Ref. 1,** p. 1461)

5. **(A)** Torsion of the spermatic cord usually occurs in adolescent males and requires urgent treatment; otherwise, it results in gangrene of the testis. (**Ref. 1,** pp. 1463–1464; **Ref. 2,** p. 1731; **Ref. 6,** p. 945)

6. **(A)** Papillary transitional cell carcinomas at the base of the bladder are best treated by transurethral resection. (**Ref. 1,** pp. 1452–1453; **Ref. 6,** p. 954)

7. **(A)** Hypernephroma is more common in men than women, is usually encapsulated, and frequently metastasizes to the lung. Tumor thrombi can extend into the renal vein and inferior vena cava. Radiotherapy is of little effect. (**Ref. 6,** p. 944–945)

8. **(B)** In the uncircumcised male, collection of smegma under the foreskin probably acts as a carcinogen, leading to increased incidence of carcinoma of the penis. Hence, it is rare in neonatally circumcised males. (**Ref. 1,** p. 1474)

9. **(C)** Retroperitoneal fibrosis surrounds the ureter, drawing it medially, and causes ureteral obstruction. (**Ref. 1,** p. 1447)

10. **(E)** The etiology of renal calculi is varied; common predisposing factors are infection, stasis in the urinary tract, and hypercalciuria. Hyperthyroidism is not a cause. All others are etiologic factors for stone formation. (**Ref. 1,** pp. 1440–1442; **Ref. 5,** p. 361)

11. **(B)** Pure uric acid stones are radiolucent. Cystine calculi are radiopaque because of their sulfur content. The others contain calcium and are radiopaque. (**Ref. 6,** p. 934)

12. **(C)** The lesion shown in Figure 4.2 is a right-sided hydronephrosis. The most common cause of unilateral hydronephrosis is a functional disorder of the pelviureteric junction. The other causes listed may occasionally produce hydronephrosis. (**Ref. 6,** p. 924)

13. **(C)** Pyeloplasty is the procedure of choice in the treatment of congenital hydronephrosis. There are various techniques of pyelo-

plasty, and the choice depends on the anatomic features. Nephrectomy is considered only when the hydronephrosis is of longstanding origin and the renal cortex has become atrophic. Nephropexy was practiced in the past but is no longer considered effective treatment. (**Ref. 6,** p. 914)

14. (**D**)   Radical prostatectomy with pelvic lymphadenectomy offers the best results for stages A and B prostatic carcinoma. (**Ref. 1,** pp. 1470–1472; **Ref. 5,** p. 349)

15. (**B**)   Urea-splitting organisms, like *P. vulgaris* and *P. aeruginosa,* predispose to the formation of triple phosphate stones. (**Ref. 6,** p. 935)

16. (**A**)   The most common manifestation of Wilms' tumor is an abdominal mass. Hematuria and pathologic fracture of bones are late features. (**Ref. 1,** p. 1179)

17. (**B**)   The most common symptom of a renal parenchymal tumor in an adult is hematuria. Abdominal mass, anemia, and hemoptysis are late features in adults. (**Ref. 1,** pp. 1443–1444; **Ref. 5,** p. 358)

18. (**B**)   The right renal vein joins the inferior vena cava and the left joins the left renal vein. Because the left testicular vein opens to the left renal vein, a left-sided hypernephroma can press on the left testicular vein or block the left testicular vein by its spread along the renal vein and produce a left-sided varicocele. (**Ref. 5,** p. 390)

19. (**C**)   The most common cause of acute retention of urine in men is benign hyperplasia of the prostate; however, in young males, prostatic abscess is the most common cause of acute retention. (**Ref. 1,** p. 1468; **Ref. 6,** p. 904)

20. (**A**)   Though a renal tumor and a cyst both produce evidence of a space-occupying lesion on excretory pyelography and nephrotomography, they can best be differentiated from one another by a CT scan or renal angiogram. CT scanning will reveal the solid nature of a tumor. On angiography, renal tumors produce abnormal vascularity and pooling of contrast in the tumor tissue. A renal

cyst is usually avascular and displaces the blood vessels around the cyst wall. (**Ref. 1,** pp. 1443–1444)

21. **(B)** Calcification within the prostate is not a feature of benign prostatic hypertrophy; the condition is known as prostatic calculi. (**Ref. 1,** p. 1468; **Ref. 5,** p. 347)

22. **(D)** In benign prostatic hypertrophy, an enlarged prostate alone is not an indication for surgery. Even though enlarged, it may be asymptomatic. (**Ref. 1,** p. 1468; **Ref. 6,** p. 927)

23. **(B)** Removal of a diverticulum requires open operation. (**Ref. 3,** pp. 1716–1717)

24. **(C)** Nephrectomy through the transabdominal approach is advisable in resection of a tumor because the renal pedicle can be approached first before mobilizing the kidney. The other advantage is the visualization of the retroperitoneal lymph nodes and the status of the opposite kidney. (**Ref. 1,** pp. 1444–1445)

25. **(D)** The most objective test for chronic prostatitis is examination of prostatic secretions obtained by gentle massage. Greater than 10 leukocytes per high-power field confirms the diagnosis. (**Ref. 1,** p. 1467; **Ref. 5,** p. 346)

26. **(C)** Bladder tumors are frequently understaged. The depth of invasion into the bladder wall correlates best with prognosis, and superficial and deep transurethral biopsy most accurately provides this information. The other listed tests may also be useful. (**Ref. 1,** pp. 1452–1453; **Ref. 5,** p. 376)

27. **(A)** Intravesical therapy of recurrent superficial tumors or carcinoma in situ is generally successful. Response rates are currently best with BCG. (**Ref. 5,** p. 932)

28. **(E)** All of the listed entities may produce the radiographic appearance of a lucent defect in the renal pelvis. Urinary cytology, ureteroscopy, ultrasonography, or CT scanning may be required to make a definite diagnosis. (**Ref. 1,** p. 1436–1437)

29. **(E)** Infertility due to varicocele generally responds well to internal spermatic vein ligation. The "stress pattern" of decreased count and motility and increased immature sperm seen on semen analysis is thought to be due to increased intrascrotal temperature. (**Ref. 1,** p. 1466)

30. **(B)** Peak flow rate on uroflow studies and the presence of trabeculation in the bladder wall on cystoscopy or IVP correlate best with bladder outlet obstruction secondary to benign prostatic hypertrophy (BPH). Elevated residual urine, particularly when associated with azotemia or recurrent infections, provides support for this diagnosis. Prostate size provides the least helpful information. (**Ref. 1,** pp. 1468–1469)

31. **(D)** The hypospadias complex commonly includes all of the listed features except upper tract anomalies. However, in very severe cases (ie, penoscrotal or perineal hypospadias with bifid scrotum), upper tract abnormalities may occur and intersex states should be considered. (**Ref. 1,** p. 1472; **Ref. 6,** p. 920)

32. **(C)** Penile self-injection with vasoactive drugs such as papaverine, regitine, or prostaglandin, or vacuum erection devices or penile prostheses would likely restore sexual function in this patient. Vascular reconstruction may also restore sexual function, but long-term results are questionable. Sexual counseling is always helpful in cases of impotence but would not produce a functional result in this case. (**Ref. 1,** p. 1475)

33. **(C)** Cancer of the prostate generally does not produce hematuria. Nearly 50% of patients present with evidence of metastatic disease—weight loss, anemia, bone pain, and neurologic deficits in the lower limbs. (**Ref. 1,** pp. 1470–1471)

34. **(B)** The most common urinary tract pathogen accounting for over 80% of cases of cystitis and pyelonephritis is *Escherichia coli*. Other gram-negative enteric bacteria account for most of the remaining 20%. (**Ref. 1,** p. 1439; **Ref. 5,** p. 370)

35. **(D)** The current treatment of choice for most 1-cm renal pelvic calculi is extracorporeal shockwave lithotripsy (ESWL). This noninvasive technique focuses small percussion shocks on the

stone and shatters it into small fragments which pass spontaneously over a period of days to weeks. The other listed methods
are either less successful or produce more morbidity. (**Ref. 1,**
p. 1441; **Ref. 5,** p. 361)

36. **(D)** Dynamic cavernosometry measures the pressure in the cor-
pus cavernosum during pharmacologically induced erection in the
evaluation of the impotent male. The other listed tests are part of
a complete urodynamic assessment of the physiologic response of
the bladder to filling and emptying, the urethral outlet resistance,
and the integrity of the external urethral sphincter. (**Ref. 5,**
p. 368)

37. **(E)** When a retrograde ureteral catheter cannot be placed, percutaneous nephrostomy under ultrasound or CT guidance often
avoids the need for open surgery. This permits immediate relief
of obstruction and improvement of renal function. (**Ref. 1,**
pp. 1441–1442)

38. **(B)** Patients with gross hematuria after blunt trauma require a
complete evaluation of their upper and lower urinary tracts. If abdominal CT scan is not planned as part of the overall assessment,
infusion pyelography will provide an excellent look at the upper
urinary tract. Urethral and bladder disruptions are well visualized
on retrograde urethrography and cystography. Cystoscopy is not
necessary and may be hazardous in the presence of bladder or
urethral rupture. (**Ref. 1,** pp. 1445–1446; **Ref. 5,** pp. 354, 369)

39. **(B)** Total renal function is determined by comparing the blood
level of various endogenous wastes (ie, creatinine, urea) to the
level of these substances in the urine. The measured excretion of
specifically administered substances such as inulin or para-amino-
hippurate (PAH) determines specific aspects of renal function. All
of the excretory tests depend on a complete urine collection for
accuracy. (**Ref. 1,** pp. 1435–1436)

40. **(E)** Fifty percent of all vesicoenteric fistulas are secondary to sigmoid diverticulitis. Colorectal tumors account for an additional
15% to 20%. Crohn's disease is associated with 10% to 15% of
these fistulas, and primary bladder malignancy is the cause of about
5% of all vesicoenteric fistulas. (**Ref. 1,** p. 1450; **Ref. 5,** p. 371)

41. (B) Stress urinary incontinence in women is due to loss of urethral closing pressure secondary to decreased pelvic floor support with subsequent shortening of total urethral length. The surgical approach consists primarily of urethral lengthening procedures which may be done transvaginally or suprapubically. Urethral closing pressure may also be enhanced by sympathomimetic agents, which increase tone in the smooth muscle of the internal sphincter, or by exercises to increase the tone of the skeletal muscle of the external sphincter. Anticholinergic medications are useful only when the incontinence is due to detrusor instability. (**Ref. 5,** p. 372)

42. (A) All of the listed techniques are common except intraperitoneal placement of the transplanted kidney. Retroperitoneal exposure of the iliac vessels is accomplished with less difficulty and less morbidity than the intraperitoneal approach. In renal transplantation in children, the graft is frequently placed intraperitoneally because of space considerations. Internal iliac artery anastomosis is preferred over external iliac unless there is significant disease of the internal iliac artery or if the contralateral internal iliac artery has been ligated during a previous transplant. (**Ref. 1,** pp. 380–381)

43. (B) Cyclosporine is a fungal derivative that was noted to have immunosuppressive properties in 1974. It was first used clinically in 1979 with good results as a single-agent immunosuppressant. It is currently used in standard therapy as a single agent or in combination with azathioprine and/or prednisone. Use has led to significant improvement in renal allograft survival. ALS and OKT-3 are usually used in the treatment of acute rejection, but are used in some centers as part of initial induction therapy. (**Ref. 1,** pp. 382–383)

44. (A) Acute cellular rejection is common during the early days or weeks after renal transplantation. Classic signs and symptoms include malaise, fever, graft tenderness and swelling, oliguria, decreased urine sodium, and hypertension. A fine-needle graft biopsy can be done to eliminate any diagnostic uncertainty. Hematuria is rare. (**Ref. 1,** p. 383)

45. (E) Complications of renal transplantation and its attendant immunosuppression are not uncommon. In addition to all of the listed problems, ureteral leaks or stenosis, acute tubular necrosis and cytomegalovirus (CMV) infections are also seen with some frequency. (**Ref. 1,** pp. 386–389)

46. (D) Ureterocele produces a cobra-head deformity. (**Ref. 2,** pp. 1772–1774; **Ref. 3,** p. 1703)

47. (A) Varicocele is common on the left side because of the anatomy; the left testicular vein drains into the renal vein. (**Ref. 1,** p. 1466)

48. (C) Spermatocele is a diverticulum usually located in the head of the epididymis. (**Ref. 1,** p. 1465)

49. (B) Congenital hydrocele is common in children. (**Ref. 1,** p. 1466)

50. (B) Seminomas are exquisitely sensitive to radiation therapy. Bulky disease may require chemotherapy. (**Ref. 1,** p. 1462; **Ref. 5,** p. 393)

51. (C) Tumors of interstitial cells of Leydig may produce precocious puberty. These are nongerminal tumors. (**Ref. 1,** p. 1462)

52. (A) Embryonal tumors, especially the yolk sac variant, are common in children. (**Ref. 1,** pp. 1462–1463)

53. (D) Choriocarcinomas are extremely invasive, with trophoblasts invading the venous system early in the course of the disease. (**Ref. 1,** p. 1463)

54. (B) Seminomas are slow-growing tumors. They comprise 40% of germ-cell tumors. (**Ref. 1,** pp. 1462–1463)

55. (B) Congenital posterior urethral valves are the most common cause of urinary tract obstruction in boys and are best diagnosed by voiding cystourethrography. They can produce severe obstructive uropathy, renal insufficiency, and urinary tract infections and require vigorous treatment. (**Ref. 6,** pp. 922–923)

56. **(D)** The ureter (metanephric duct) develops as a hollow outgrowth (ureteric bud) from the inferior end of the mesonephric duct. An accessory ureteral bud may develop from the mesonephric duct, thereby forming a duplicated ureter. (**Ref. 1,** p. 1435)

57. **(A)** Interstitial cystitis is a urinary bladder syndrome of unknown etiology, characterized by lower abdominal pain and irritative voiding symptoms, that predominantly affects females. Submucosal glomerulations may be seen cystoscopically after hydrodistention. Therapy may consist of bladder dilatations and instillations of dimethyl sulfoxide (DMSO) and oxychlorosene. (**Ref. 5,** pp. 370–371)

58. **(C)** Congenital adrenal hyperplasia with excessive production of virilizing steroid precursors results from one of several basic enzymatic defects in the gland. It most commonly affects females and may be associated with a severe salt-losing tendency due to impaired aldosterone synthesis. (**Ref. 6,** p. 736)

6

Plastic and Reconstructive Surgery
Gregory H. Croll

DIRECTIONS (Questions 1 through 20) Each of the questions or incomplete statements below is followed by five suggested answers or completions. Select the ONE that is best in each case.

Questions 1 through 7

1. A 62-year-old man sustained an electrical injury by contact with a high-voltage power line. He has full-thickness skin loss on his thumb as shown in Figure 6.1. Initial management should be
   A. conservative debridement and immediate skin grafting
   B. amputation of the thumb to avoid systemic complications
   C. fluid resuscitation and monitoring urine output/pH
   D. immediate debridement and flap coverage
   E. urgent fasciotomies of the hand and forearm compartments

2. Acceptable reconstructive options for the postmastectomy patient shown in Figure 6.2 include
   A. placement of a tissue expander and subsequent exchange for a permanent saline-filled prosthesis

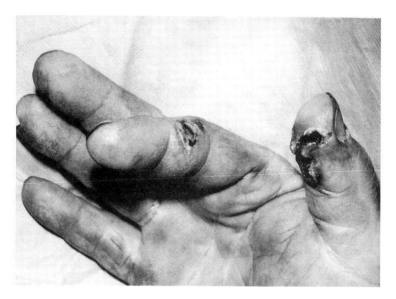

Figure 6.1

   B. free tissue transfer with a transverse rectus abdominis myo-
cutaneous flap
   C. no reconstruction
   D. pedicled rectus abdominis myocutaneous flap
   E. all of the above

3. A 21-year-old male falls on his outstretched right hand while
playing basketball. He comes in two days later and has pain in the
radial side of the wrist and is very tender to palpation dorsally
distal to the radial styloid. X-rays are read as "negative" for fracture. Initial management of this patient should be to
   A. suggest that he avoid strenuous use of this hand for 4 to 7
days, take anti-inflammatory medication, and gradually return to normal activities
   B. immobilize the wrist in a splint for 4 to 7 days and repeat x-ray
   C. immobilize the wrist/thumb in a thumb spica splint or cast
for 14 days, reexamine patient, and repeat x-ray
   D. repair or refer patient for repair of radial collateral ligament
   E. since there is no significant injury, no treatment is needed;
instruct patient to return if it doesn't improve in 7 days

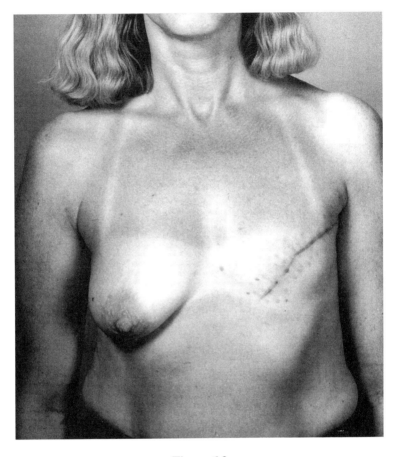

Figure 6.2

4. All of the following are compressive neuropathies potentially involving the median nerve EXCEPT
   A. pronator syndrome
   B. posterior interosseous syndrome
   C. carpal tunnel syndrome
   D. anterior interosseous syndrome
   E. cervical root compression

5. First and second branchial arch syndrome can include all of the following EXCEPT
   A. external ear anomalies
   B. macrostomia
   C. absence of the parotid gland
   D. colobomata
   E. mandibular hypoplasia

6. The "Allen's Test" evaluates the patency of
   A. ulnar artery
   B. radial artery
   C. superficial palmar arch
   D. radial and ulnar arteries
   E. radial and ulnar arteries and the superficial palmar arch

7. Which of the following would be BEST treated by Mohs' chemo-surgery?
   A. 2-cm diameter melanoma of the back
   B. subungual acral lentiginous melanoma
   C. nodular basal cell carcinoma of the malar area
   D. morphemic basal cell carcinoma of the medial canthus
   E. squamous cell carcinoma of the lower lip

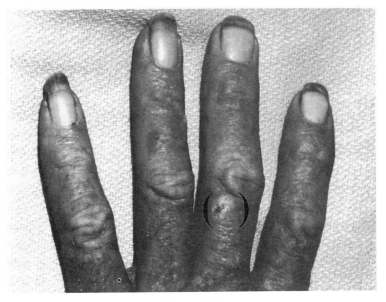

Figure 6.3

Questions 8 and 9

A 74-year-old farmer gives a history of this 7-mm diameter by 5-mm high lesion on the dorsum of his long finger (see Figure 6.3). It had been present for approximately 6 to 8 weeks and growing very rapidly. Its center recently became depressed and ulcerated.

8. The MOST likely diagnosis is
   A. basal cell carcinoma
   B. nodular melanoma
   C. acral lentiginous melanoma
   D. keratoacanthoma
   E. actinic keratosis

9. Of the following choices, the BEST management would be
   A. digital amputation
   B. ray amputation
   C. irradiation and excision of any remaining lesion
   D. observation
   E. isolated hyperthermic limb perfusion

Questions 10 through 20

10. Malocclusion can be seen in which of the following?
    A. subcondylar mandible fracture
    B. LeFort III fracture
    C. LeFort I fracture
    D. displaced zygoma fracture
    E. all of the above

11. A 39-year-old female presents with a painless mass in the soft tissue overlying the angle of the jaw. The mass has been present for at least four years. The MOST likely diagnosis is
    A. adenoid cystic carcinoma
    B. Warthin's tumor
    C. mucoepidermoid carcinoma
    D. pleomorphic adenoma
    E. parotitis

12. The muscle that abducts the index finger is the
    A. second lumbrical
    B. first dorsal interosseous
    C. second volar interosseus
    D. first lumbrical
    E. second dorsal interosseus

13. All of the following are common complaints or findings in carpal tunnel syndrome EXCEPT
    A. numbness in the thumb
    B. numbness that awakens the patient at night
    C. numbness in the palm
    D. positive Phalen's test
    E. symptoms aggravated by activity

14. Dupuytren's contracture
    A. is a common sequela of severe burns
    B. is a result of failure-to-decompress compartment syndrome
    C. is caused by contracture of the tendon(s)
    D. is a disease of the palmar fascia
    E. routinely implies a poor prognosis for hand function

15. Motor innervation of the orbicularis oris muscle is by
  A. mental nerve
  B. inferior alveolar nerve
  C. marginal mandibular branch of cranial nerve VII
  D. buccal branch of cranial nerve VII
  E. infraorbital nerve

16. The earliest visible indication of oral squamous cell carcinoma in situ is
  A. a submucosal mass
  B. a lichen planus
  C. leukoplakia
  D. a nodular lesion with irregular pearly borders
  E. persistent erythema

17. Toxic shock syndrome following rhinoplasty is most commonly associated with
  A. cartilage grafting
  B. external approach
  C. bone grafting
  D. nasal packing
  E. intranasal splints

18. Successful "take" of a full-thickness or split-thickness skin graft depends upon all of the following EXCEPT
  A. complete fixation
  B. maintained immobilization
  C. firm but not excessive pressure
  D. clean, white fascia beneath the graft
  E. absence of blood clot beneath the graft

19. Which of the following is NOT associated with an increased incidence of carcinoma of the lip?
  A. lower lip location
  B. female gender
  C. light-colored skin
  D. chronic irritation
  E. tobacco exposure

20. A cystic hygroma
   A.   is a unilocular cyst
   B.   is found most often in the mediastinum
   C.   is usually seen in infants and young children
   D.   often undergoes malignant transformation
   E.   should be treated with radiation therapy

Plastic and Reconstructive Surgery

Answers and Comments

1. (C) Electrical injuries can be deceptively extensive. Aside from the obvious local injury, there is often extensive distant injury (neurologic, vascular, and muscular). The zone of obvious injury frequently enlarges to a significantly greater area over the first 7 to 14 days following the injury. Tissue that appears graftable (and, indeed, may well support a graft initially) frequently progresses to necrosis. It is the knowledge of this natural history of electrical injuries that makes most surgeons cautious about very early coverage of wounds. While occasionally necessary to avoid compressive injury to deep tissues, fasciotomies should not be done routinely, but certainly the need for them must be constantly kept in mind. Likewise, amputations should not be a routine procedure but may need to be done as the tissue necrosis or functional loss dictates. The extensive injury frequently causes myonecrosis, and urine should routinely be checked for myoglobin; if present, fluid resuscitation should be aggressive to maintain a good urine output and the urine alkalinized to minimize the precipitation in the kidney and resultant renal insufficiency. (**Ref. 1,** pp. 195–196)

2. (E) Since the choice of whether or not to undergo breast reconstruction is a matter of personal preference of the patient, *no* reconstruction certainly is a reasonable option. While there may be certain factors affecting the choice of reconstructive technique (ie, patient/surgeon preference, previous abdominal incisions, overall patient condition, etc.), all of the above listed techniques are acceptable options. (**Ref. 1,** pp. 551–552; **Ref. 2,** p. 2062)

3. **(C)** This case represents the classic history of a scaphoid fracture. The fracture is notorious for its delayed appearance radiographically. It is for both clinical and medicolegal reasons that patients with this history and physical presentation (ie, pain in the "anatomic snuff box") must be immobilized when initially seen and then reexamined clinically and radiographically, usually in two weeks. It is helpful if scaphoid views are specifically requested with the wrist films. If a scaphoid fracture is found and is nondisplaced, cast immobilization for eight weeks (frequently longer) is needed. If displaced, surgical intervention with internal fixation may be necessary. Missed fractures result in chronically painful conditions which limit wrist motion. (**Ref. 1,** pp. 1309–1310; **Ref. 2,** p. 1917)

4. **(B)** The posterior interosseous nerve is the motor terminal branch of the *radial* nerve. The median nerve can be compressed in multiple locations from its cervical roots, distally by the lacertus fibrosis, pronator teres on the proximal arch of the flexor digitorum superficialis (pronator syndrome). The anterior interosseous syndrome (multiple causes) usually involves forearm pain and weakness or paralysis of the flexor pollicis longus. Carpal tunnel syndrome (the most common form of median nerve compression) involves the branches of the median nerve which course under the transverse carpal ligament. (**Ref. 1,** pp. 1370–1372)

5. **(D)** Colobomata are congenital clefts in the eyelid associated with a variety of craniofacial syndromes, the most common of which is Treacher–Collins syndrome. Eyelids are not derivatives of the first and second branchial arches; first and second branchial arch syndrome (hemifacial microsomia) can involve any of the structures derived from these arches. In addition to the deformities listed, underdevelopment of the zygoma and temporal bone are common. (**Ref. 1,** p. 1226; **Ref. 2,** p. 2045)

6. **(E)** Allen's test is used to assess the vascular supply of the hand. With both ulnar and radial arteries occluded above the wrist, the patient actively exsanguinates the hand by making and releasing a fist several times. One artery is released and the opposite side of the hand is checked for refill (eg, radial artery release, check *ulnar* side of hand). If the entire hand fills, both the open artery and the palmar arch are patent. If only the ipsilateral side fills (e.g. radial, in this example), the test artery is patent and the arch is not. If no refill occurs, the test vessel is occluded. The test is then repeated reversing the vessel that is not occluded. (**Ref. 2,** p. 490)

7. **(D)** Mohs' chemosurgery was developed to allow the ablative surgeon to be able to assess the margins of excision as the lesion is being excised. Its best uses are for difficult lesions situated in critical areas (ie, eyelids, canthal areas, nose, etc.) where the *least* amount of excision that will provide adequate margin is needed. Morpheic basal cell carcinomata are notorious for their treacherously infiltrative spread and high recurrence rate. A morpheic basal cell in the medial canthal region is an excellent situation in which to utilize the Mohs' technique. All of the other lesions described can be handled quite well with standard surgical excision with frozen section and/or permanent pathology control. (**Ref. 2,** pp. 523–524)

8. **(D)** See answer 9 comments.

9. **(D)** The history and appearance of this lesion are those of a classic keratoacanthoma. Without the history, it is conceivable that this *could* be a basal cell carcinoma, malignant melanoma, or acral lentiginous melanoma. Actinic keratoses typically are erythematous and/or scaly plaques on sun-exposed skin. A keratoacanthoma typically regresses by approximately 6 months after its appearance, often leaving only a small scar. Therefore, observation is a reasonable choice. (However, due to their appearance, they are frequently excised. There remains controversy among pathologists as to whether these lesions are benign or represent very well-differentiated squamous cell carcinoma). None of the other treatment options are appropriate for a keratoacanthoma. (**Ref. 1,** p. 1390)

10. **(E)** Malocclusion (improper occlusion of the maxillary and mandibular teeth) can occur in several types of injuries. LeFort fractures separate the maxillary arch from its normal alignment with the skull base, thereby usually causing malocclusion with the mandibular dentition. Any fracture of the mandible tends to cause some degree of malocclusion. While the zygoma itself is separate from the tooth-bearing maxillary arch, *displaced* zygoma fractures frequently impinge on the coronoid process of the mandible, causing trismus and malocclusion. (**Ref. 5,** pp. 145–152)

11. **(D)** The most common parotid tumor is the benign pleomorphic adenoma (mixed tumor). It is more common in females and represents approximately 65% of all salivary tumors and 80% of all benign salivary tumors. Approximately 10% will undergo malignant degeneration. Warthin's tumor (papillary cystadenoma lymphomatosum) is also a benign salivary tumor found only in the parotid. It is much less common, as are mucoepidermoid and adenoid cystic carcinoma. Only approximately 15% of parotid tumors are malignant with mucoepidermoid being the most common in the parotid and adenoid cystic being the most common in the submandibular glands. (**Ref. 1,** p. 1232)

12. **(B)** If the function of the first dorsal interosseous muscle is remembered (ie, *ab*duction of the index finger), the function of all of the other interossei can be deduced (ie, the three volar interossei adduct the digits to the third ray). The lumbricals contribute to flexion of the metacarpal phalangeal (MP) joints and extension of the interphalangeal (IP) joints through contribution to the lateral bands. (**Ref. 1,** p. 1314)

13. **(C)** The palmar cutaneous nerve of the median nerve usually branches several centimeters above the transverse carpal ligament and passes superficial to this to enter the palm. Therefore, numbness in the palm suggests a higher site of compression (ie, pronator syndrome). Carpal tunnel syndrome may coexist with pronator syndrome ("double crush" phenomenon). The other choices are all common in carpal tunnel syndrome. (**Ref. 2,** pp. 2010–2011)

14. **(D)** Dupuytren's contracture is a disease of the palmar fascia. Progressive fibrosis causes the classic nodules and skin puckering, as well as joint contractures. When minimally symptomatic

and without functional loss, most hand surgeons are conservative in their recommendations for surgical intervention. Metacarpophalangeal joint contractures can be present for extended periods (ie, months to even years) and will usually do well if and when released and the diseased fascia excised. However, interphalangeal joint contractures must be addressed early (ie, weeks) after occurrence to avoid significant collateral ligament shortening and joint stiffness. Tendons are not involved in the Dupuytren's disease process. Volkmann's (ischemic) contracture can be a result of failure-to-decompress compartment syndrome. While burns frequently cause scar contracture, they do not cause Dupuytren's contracture. (**Ref. 2,** pp. 2012–2013)

15. **(D)**   Of the choices listed, three (A, B, and E) are purely sensory. The inferior alveolar nerve enters the mandible medially and exits anteriorly below the canine as the mental nerve, which gives sensory innervation to the lower lip. The infraorbital nerve provides sensation to the upper lip and medial cheek. The buccal branch of the facial nerve innervates the elevators of the lip and the orbicularis oris. The marginal mandibular branch of the facial nerve innervates the depressors of the mouth. (**Ref. 5,** pp. 144–152)

16. **(E)**   A large prospective study has confirmed that erythroplasia is the earliest visible warning sign of oral cancer. In a group of over 500 tobacco users who had asymptomatic lesions, 60% had red lesions and 14% had white ones (leukoplakia). Lichen planus is characterized by lacy white lesions. Leukoplakia represents hyperkeratosis from chronic inflammation, not necessarily malignant or dysplastic. Submucosal masses are more likely salivary gland tumors or mucous cysts. A nodular lesion with pearly borders is most characteristic of a basal cell carcinoma. (**Ref. 2,** p. 604)

17. **(D)**   Toxic shock syndrome consists of sudden onset of high fever, hypotension, diarrhea, and erythredema. A *Staphylococcus aureus*-produced toxin is believed to be causative. When associated with rhinoplasty, prolonged (greater than 3 days) nasal packing has been associated with most cases. This seems to provide an environment most suitable to bacterial overgrowth. A very small number of cases have been reported with the use of intranasal

splints. Cartilage grafting, bone grafting, and an external surgical approach have not been found to be related. (**Ref. 2,** p. 519; **Ref. 5,** p. 188)

18. **(D)**   Successful appropriation of a new blood supply by grafted skin ("take") depends upon all of the items except a clean fascia bed. Such a bed does not usually possess the vascular supply to support the graft. (**Ref. 1,** p. 1386)

19. **(B)**   Females do not have a higher incidence of lip cancer; 87% occur in males. (**Ref. 1,** p. 1217)

20. **(C)**   Cystic hygroma is a malformation involving lymphatics. It is usually seen in the necks of young children. It does not undergo malignant change and should be treated by excision, not radiation. (**Ref. 1,** pp. 1176–1177)

7

Otolaryngology
Paul R. Cook

DIRECTIONS (Questions 1 through 18): Each of the questions or incomplete statements below is followed by five suggested answers or completions. Select the ONE that is best in each case.

1. Regarding laryngeal cancer, which of the following is FALSE?
    A. hoarseness appears early
    B. involved nodes are not palpable in 35% of cases
    C. distant metastasis appears early
    D. direct extension is common
    E. it is 90% five-year curable when limited to one cord

2. All of the following are removed in radical neck dissection EXCEPT the
    A. sternocleidomastoid muscle
    B. external carotid artery
    C. internal jugular vein
    D. spinal accessory nerve
    E. submaxillary gland

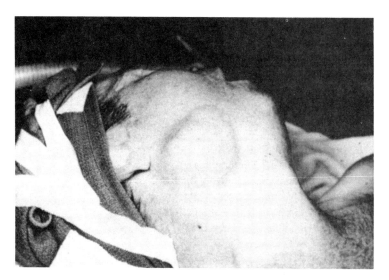

Figure 7.1

3. Which of the following factors is NOT associated with squamous cell carcinoma of the larynx?
   A. male sex
   B. age in fifth and sixth decades
   C. history of woodworking
   D. large ethanol intake
   E. tobacco smoking

4. A 16-year-old male presents with a 3-cm nontender fluctuant mass in the right jugulodigastric area anterior to the sternocleido-mastoid muscle (Figure 7.1). The MOST likely diagnosis is
   A. ectopic thyroid
   B. branchial cleft cyst
   C. thyroglossal duct cyst
   D. sebaceous cyst
   E. pharyngeal fistula

5. In LeFort I fractures, the fragment consists of all of the following EXCEPT the
   A. upper teeth and palate
   B. lower portions of the pterygoid processes
   C. portions of the walls of both maxillary antra
   D. nasal spine
   E. bridge of the nose

6. In general, traumatic perforations of the tympanic membrane
   A. are a surgical emergency
   B. will heal spontaneously in most cases
   C. usually require operative repair
   D. require microsurgical repair
   E. require a graft for repair

7. The MOST common organism in acute otitis media of older children and adults is
   A. *Staphylococcus*
   B. *Streptococcus*
   C. *Hemophilus influenzae*
   D. *Klebsiella pneumoniae*
   E. *Pseudomonas*

8. The incidence of cervical spine injuries with significant facial fractures is
   A. 7%
   B. 12%
   C. 23%
   D. 46%
   E. 55%

9. A 65-year-old white male who has been smoking pipes since early adulthood notes a small patch of white on the lateral anterior portion of the tongue. The patch is not painful for the first month, but gradually becomes more painful as it begins to enlarge and ulcerate. The MOST likely diagnosis is
   A. benign nonspecific ulceration
   B. leukoplakia (benign)
   C. epulis
   D. carcinoma of the tongue
   E. ranula of the tongue

10. The diagnosis in question 9 may be confirmed by
    A. a positive Wasserman test
    B. a positive lupus erythematosus (LE) preparation
    C. a biopsy of the lesion
    D. diagnostic mandibular and maxillary x-rays
    E. observation of further progression of the disease

11. A cholesteatoma is
    A. an atherosclerotic lesion
    B. a dermal collection of cholesterol salts
    C. epithelial debris in the middle ear
    D. a yellow papule beneath the oral tongue
    E. retained cerumen

12. Small, malignant tumors of the larynx that are intrinsic in origin
    and have not spread beyond the larynx are BEST treated by
    A. irradiation
    B. laryngofissure
    C. total laryngectomy
    D. total laryngectomy and radical neck dissection
    E. radium needle implants

13. The basic pathology in MOST cases of prominent ears is
    A. hypertrophy of the ear
    B. failure of mesodermal penetration
    C. lack of development of the antihelix
    D. hypoplasia of the extrinsic ear musculature
    E. gigantism

14. Clinical features of facial fractures frequently include all of the
    following EXCEPT
    A. deformity
    B. facial nerve paralysis
    C. anesthesia over areas of trigeminal branch distribution
    D. ocular disparity
    E. malocclusion of the teeth

15. The MOST sensitive test for nasal fracture is
  - **A.** history
  - **B.** physical diagnosis
  - **C.** plain x-ray studies
  - **D.** magnetic resonance imaging
  - **E.** computed tomography (CT) scanning

16. Mixed tumors of the salivary gland
  - **A.** are most common in the submaxillary gland
  - **B.** are usually malignant
  - **C.** are most common in the parotid gland
  - **D.** usually cause facial paralysis
  - **E.** are associated with calculi

17. In epistaxis, what percentage of the cases will respond to ten minutes of direct pressure?
  - **A.** 10%
  - **B.** 30%
  - **C.** 70%
  - **D.** 90%
  - **E.** 0%

18. Choanal atresia is a severe risk for newborns because of
  - **A.** abdominal distention
  - **B.** coexistent vascular malformations
  - **C.** resulting inadequate respiration
  - **D.** associated enzyme abnormalities
  - **E.** associated renal abnormalities

DIRECTIONS (Questions 19 through 21): The group of questions below consists of lettered headings followed by a list of numbered words, phrases, or statements. For each numbered word, phrase, or statement, select the ONE lettered heading that is most closely associated with it. Each lettered heading may be used once, more than once, or not at all.

Questions 19 through 21

Match the respective nasal meatus in the questions below with the appropriate lettered choice from the list below. See Figures 7.2A (view from mid-palate with turbinates intact) and 7.2B (same view with turbinates partially removed).

   A. ostium of the sphenoid sinus
   B. ostium of the maxillary sinus
   C. nasal lacrimal duct
   D. sinus lateralis ostium

19. Superior meatus

20. Middle meatus

21. Inferior meatus

DIRECTIONS (Questions 22 through 40): Each of the questions or incomplete statements below is followed by five suggested answers or completions. Select the ONE that is best in each case.

22. Which of the following is NOT a cause for conductive hearing loss?
   A. otitis media
   B. otosclerosis
   C. noise-induced hearing loss
   D. perforation of the tympanic membrane
   E. ossicular chain disruption

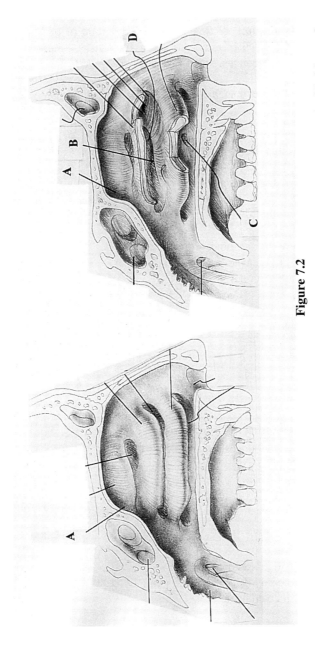

Figure 7.2

From Bailey, Byron J., Johnson, Jonas T., Kohut, Robert I., Pillsbury, Harold C., Tardy, Eugene M., Jr. (eds.): *Head and Neck Surgery—Otolaryngology*, p. 343, Figures 27.1 and 27.2, Philadelphia, J.B. Lippincott Company, 1993.

23. Conductive hearing losses are usually reversible. Which of the following conditions is reversible by surgical treatment?
   A. otosclerosis
   B. presbycusis
   C. sudden hearing loss
   D. ototoxicity
   E. meningitis

24. What is the BEST treatment for most cases of sensorineural hearing loss associated with aging (presbycusis)?
   A. nothing
   B. hearing aid
   C. ear trumpet
   D. diuretic therapy
   E. labyrinthectomy

25. The MOST common benign lesion of the external ear is
   A. melanoma
   B. chondrodermatitis nodularis chronicus helicus
   C. cerumenoma
   D. actinic keratosis
   E. exostosis of the canal

26. MOST of the infectious and/or inflammatory diseases involving the middle ear space are secondary to
   A. ciliary dyskinesia
   B. resistant pathogens
   C. eustachian tube dysfunction
   D. tobacco abuse
   E. allergic diathesis

27. Acute otitis is
   A. a rare condition
   B. the most common reason ill children visit the doctor
   C. usually not accompanied by pain and fever
   D. caused by coliform bacteria
   E. treated by placing ventilating tubes

28. A 5-year-old child has persistent serous effusions in both ears for 6 months after a routine acute infection. He has a 40-dB conductive hearing loss in both ears and has been having trouble in school. What would be the BEST treatment for this child?

    A. observe the child for another 3 months

    B. prescribe amoxicillin for 10 days

    C. recommend hearing aids

    D. place ventilating tubes

    E. prescribe prophylactic antibiotics for 3 months

29. A 3-year-old child has had eight episodes of acute otitis media in 6 months and has difficulty resolving the effusions between infections. What should be done to effectively eliminate the infections?

    A. continue treating each infection as it arises

    B. place ventilating tubes

    C. prescribe prophylactic antibiotics for 6 months

    D. remove the tonsils

    E. give IV antibiotics for 4 weeks after infectious disease consultation

30. The following clinical entities are common causes for tinnitus EXCEPT

    A. high-frequency hearing loss

    B. Ménière's disease

    C. ototoxic drugs

    D. loud noise exposure

    E. acute otitis media

31. Vertigo is very common in all of the following conditions EXCEPT

    A. vestibular neuritis

    B. Ménière's disease

    C. presbycusis

    D. viral labyrinthitis

    E. benign paroxysmal positional vertigo

32. Which of the following is the MOST common anatomic deformity causing nasal obstruction (see Figure 7.3)?

    A. septal deviation

    B. foreign bodies

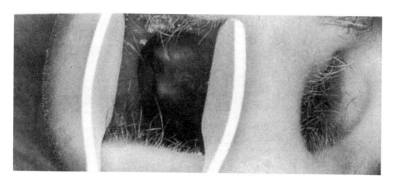

Figure 7.3

From Bull, T.R.: *A Color Atlas of E.N.T. Diagnosis,* 2nd ed., p. 123, Figure 211, London, Wolfe Medical Publications Ltd., 1992.

    C. septal hematoma from nasal fracture
    D. nasal polyps
    E. hypertrophic nasal turbinates

33. Which of the following is the MOST common infectious disease in man?
    A. acute otitis media
    B. acute viral rhinitis
    C. viral pharyngitis
    D. acute gastroenteritis
    E. mycoplasma pneumonia

34. A 20-year-old white male presents with paroxysmal sneezing, nasal itching and obstruction, and copious clear rhinorrhea. On physical exam, you note pale bluish nasal mucosa and thin, clear nasal secretions. He only has these symptoms during the spring and fall. What is the MOST likely diagnosis?
    A. viral rhinitis
    B. vasomotor rhinitis
    C. seasonal allergic rhintis
    D. chemical sensitivity (irritant rhinitis)
    E. perennial allergic rhinitis

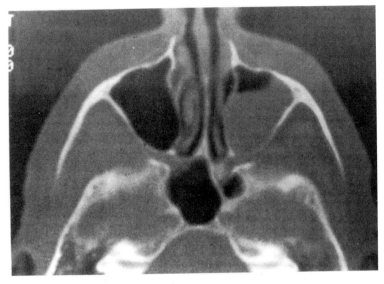

Figure 7.4

From Lee, K.J. (ed.): *Textbook of Otolaryngology and Head and Neck Surgery,* p. 267, Figure 15.58, New York, Elsevier, 1989.

35. Which of the following pathogens is MOST likely to cause acute sinusitis, as shown in Figure 7.4?

   A. *Staphylococcus aureus*
   B. *Pseudomonas aeruginosa*
   C. *Streptococcus pneumoniae*
   D. *Streptococcus pyogenes*
   E. *Bacteroides melanogenicus*

36. All of the following are indications for tonsillectomy EXCEPT

   A. six to seven episodes of tonsillitis in 1 year
   B. airway obstruction secondary to tonsillar hypertrophy
   C. repeat ear and sinus infections
   D. recurrent peritonsillar abscess
   E. very large asymmetric tonsil in an adult

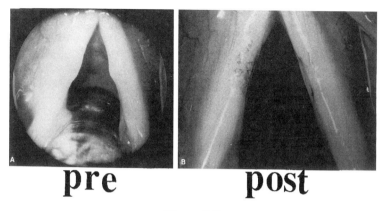

Figure 7.5

From Bailey, Byron J., Johnson, Jonas T., Kohut, Robert I., Pillsbury, Harold C., Tardy, Eugene M., Jr. (eds.): *Head and Neck Surgery–Otolaryngoly,* p. 633, Figure 50.3, Philadelphia, J.B. Lippincott Company, 1993.

37. The MOST common cause for infant stridor, accounting for 60% of the cases, is
   A. subglottic hemangioma
   B. vocal cord paralysis
   C. laryngomalacia
   D. congenital webs
   E. laryngeal cleft

38. The treatment of choice for vocal cord nodules (singer's nodes), shown in Figure 7.5A (pretreatment) and 7.5B (posttreatment) is
   A. psychotherapy
   B. vocal cord stripping
   C. vocal rehabilitation (speech therapy)
   D. no treatment necessary
   E. microlaryngoscopy with laser ablation of the nodules

39. What is the MOST common cause of acquired subglottic stenosis?
   A. motor vehicular trauma
   B. prolonged endotracheal intubation
   C. chronic bronchitis
   D. tracheoesophageal fistula
   E. previous tracheal surgery

40. The fastest, safest means of establishing a surgical airway is
   A. endoscopic intubation
   B. tracheotomy under local anesthesia
   C. tracheotomy under general anesthesia
   D. cricothyrotomy
   E. puncture through the thyrohyoid membrane

Otolaryngology

Answers and Comments

1. (C) Metastases from laryngeal carcinoma are usually late, and the disease is usually confined to the larynx. (**Ref. 1,** pp. 1206–1207; **Ref. 2,** pp. 601–602)

2. (B) In radical neck dissection, the carotid artery and its branches are not removed. On the other hand, for the complete removal of lymph nodes and draining areas, it is essential to remove the sternocleidomastoid muscle, internal jugular vein, submaxillary gland, and spinal accessory nerve. (**Ref. 1,** p. 1223; **Ref. 2,** pp. 616–618)

3. (C) History of woodworking is not associated with squamous cell carcinoma of the larynx. (**Ref. 1,** pp. 1206–1207; **Ref. 2,** p. 600)

4. (B) This is a typical branchial cleft cyst. These cysts are usually located along the anterior border of the sternocleidomastoid muscle. Ranula is a cyst under the tongue; thyroglossal cysts are located between the chin and the laryngeal cartilage; and epulis is fibrous hyperplasia of the gingiva. Sebaceous cysts can appear anywhere and are not specifically situated in the lateral neck. (**Ref. 2,** p. 596)

5. (E) In LeFort I fracture, the fragment consists of the hard palate, the alveolar margin including the teeth, the lower portion of the pterygoid processes, portions of both maxillary antra, and the nasal spine. It does not include the bridge of the nose. (**Ref. 1,** p. 288)

6. **(B)** Most perforations (90%) will heal spontaneously within 6 weeks. (**Ref. 1,** p. 1189; **Ref. 5,** p. 183)

7. **(B)** *Streptococcus* infections are most common in the age group over 8 years of age. (**Ref. 1,** p. 1190)

8. **(A)** Approximately 7% of all patients with major fractures of the upper and lower jaws have injuries of the cervical spine. (**Ref. 1,** pp. 282–283)

9. **(D)** Carcinoma of the tongue is the most likely lesion, because it is ulcerated and has changed in character from what it was before. The long history of smoking and the history suggestive of leukoplakia are predisposing factors. (**Ref. 1,** p. 1221; **Ref. 2,** pp. 605–610)

10. **(C)** Biopsy of the lesion is the best method of confirming the diagnosis. A number of these patients have positive serology, but this does not always indicate previous syphilitic infections. X-rays are of no value in the early stages, and observation without tissue diagnosis should not be practiced. (**Ref. 1,** p. 1224)

11. **(C)** Cholesteatoma occurs when the middle ear becomes lined with stratified squamous epithelium, which then desquamates in the closed space. This occurs secondary to perforations in the pars flaccida with ingrowth of squamous epithelium from the outer canal. (**Ref. 1,** p. 1192).

12. **(A)** Intrinsic localized tumors of the larynx are best treated by irradiation. Larger, higher-staged tumors need combined therapy. Survival in early lesions is excellent. (**Ref. 1,** p. 1207; **Ref. 2,** p. 613)

13. **(C)** The basic deformity in prominent ears is lack of development of the antihelical fold. (**Ref. 1,** p. 1193; **Ref. 2,** p. 2055)

14. **(B)** Facial fractures do not usually involve paralysis of the facial nerve. Impaired muscular contraction is due to pain. Facial

nerve injuries occur in fractures of the temporal bone. (**Ref. 2,** pp. 2058–2059)

15. **(B)** The gold standard in the diagnosis and treatment of nasal fractures is physical diagnosis revealing nasal deformity and palpable step-off. Deviation of the cartilaginous septum may be secondary to the trauma. Septal hematoma must be ruled out by direct examination. Radiographs are generally of little value. (**Ref. 1,** p. 1196; **Ref. 2,** pp. 2052–2053)

16. **(C)** The most common site of mixed tumors of the salivary gland is the parotid. The majority of them are benign, and facial paralysis is very uncommon. (**Ref. 1,** p. 1232; **Ref. 2,** pp. 650–651)

17. **(D)** Ninety percent of nosebleeds occur in the plexus of vessels in the anterior–inferior part of the septum. These will respond to digital pressure for 10 minutes. The remainder of cases of epistaxis will require posterior packing or more aggressive management. (**Ref. 1,** p. 1197)

18. **(C)** Newborns are obligate nose breathers such that children with choanal atresia are only able to breathe during crying. If this is not diagnosed and treated expeditiously, respiratory distress will ensue. (**Ref. 1,** p. 1199)

19. **(A)** The ostia of the posterior ethmoid cells and the sphenoid ostium are in the superior meatus. (**Ref. 1,** p. 1195)

20. **(B)** The ostia of the anterior ethmoid cells, the maxillary sinuses, and the frontal duct open into the middle meatus. (**Ref. 1,** p. 1195)

21. **(C)** The nasolacrimal duct opens into the inferior meatus. (**Ref. 1,** p. 1195)

22. **(C)** Noise-induced hearing loss is sensorineural. All of the other causes listed are characterized by conductive losses. (**Ref. 5,** p. 179)

23. **(A)** Otosclerosis, which causes fixation of the stapes footplate and a conductive loss, is the correct answer. The other answers are associated with sensorineural losses. (**Ref. 5,** p. 179)

24. **(B)** Most cases of presbycusis can be remediated with amplification. The best method is by using a modern hearing aid. In the past, an ear trumpet did help somewhat. (**Ref. 5,** pp. 179, 183)

25. **(D)** Actinic keratosis (AK) is the best answer. The other conditions listed are considerably more rare. AKs are best treated by removal. (**Ref. 5,** pp. 180–181)

26. **(C)** The eustachian tube is the only drainage and ventilation organ for the middle ear. It is a dynamic structure and can be compromised by mucosal edema caused by various inflammatory conditions. The other responses are factors in the pathogenesis of eustachian tube dysfunction. (**Ref. 5,** p. 182)

27. **(B)** This is the most common reason for sick children visits to primary care physicians. The disease is usually characterized by pain and fever. The most common pathogens are *S. pneumoniae* and *H. influenzae,* not coliforms. Antibiotics are the treatment of choice. Placement of ventilating tubes is reserved for cases that are refractory to antibiotics or are multiply occurring. (**Ref. 5,** p. 182)

28. **(D)** This scenario highlights one of the primary indications for ventilating tube placement. The other management choices are inappropriate. (**Ref. 5,** p. 182)

29. **(B)** This is the other primary reason for placing ventilating tubes. The other options will not eliminate the cyclical pattern of infections and retained fluid. (**Ref. 5,** p. 182)

30. **(E)** High-frequency losses, Ménière's disease, ototoxic drugs, and loud noise exposure are all associated with tinnitus (ringing). Acute otitis media is not associated with tinnitus. (**Ref. 5,** pp. 183–184)

31. (C) Presbycusis is not commonly associated with vertigo; the other diseases listed are. (**Ref. 5,** pp. 183–184)

32. (A) Septal deviation is the correct response. The other conditions are causes of nasal obstruction but are less common. (**Ref. 5,** pp. 187–189)

33. (B) Acute viral rhinitis, or the common cold, is caused by a variety of viruses. It has the highest prevalence in children under 5 years. The other diseases listed are less common. (**Ref. 5,** pp. 189–190)

34. (C) This is the typical presentation for an individual suffering from seasonal allergic rhinitis. The fact that the young man has these symptoms only in the spring and fall makes allergic rhinitis the most likely diagnosis. (**Ref. 5,** p. 190)

35. (C) *Streptococcus pneumoniae, Hemophilus influenzae,* and *Moraxella catarrhalis* are the most common pathogens in acute sinusitis. *Staphylococcus aureus* is a common pathogen in *chronic* sinusitis. The other pathogens would be rare in the pathogenesis of acute sinusitis. (**Ref. 5,** pp. 191–193)

36. (C) There is no evidence that tonsillectomy for ear and sinus disease has any merit. The other responses constitute the primary indications for tonsillectomy. (**Ref. 5,** pp. 194–195)

37. (C) Laryngomalacia, or soft, floppy larynx, is the most common cause of infant stridor, accounting for 60% of all cases. It presents as high-pitched inspiratory stridor that worsens in the supine position. The other conditions listed are less common. (**Ref. 5,** pp. 198–199)

38. (C) Vocal rehabilitation is the first and best therapy for vocal cord nodules. Laser ablation should be reserved for recalcitrant cases. Cord stripping is too severe and may result in greater hoarseness. (**Ref. 5,** pp. 199–200)

39. (B) By far, the most common cause of acquired subglottic stenosis is prolonged endotracheal intubation. In older children and adults, a tracheotomy should be considered after 7 to 10 days of intubation. (**Ref. 5,** p. 200)

40. (D) Cricothyrotomy is currently the standard of care and is recommended by the American College of Surgeons and the American Academy of Otolaryngology–Head and Neck Surgery. Endoscopic intubation is not a surgical airway. (**Ref. 5,** p. 200)

8

Neurosurgery
John J. Oro
Scott R. Gibbs

DIRECTIONS (Questions 1 through 11): Each of the questions or incomplete statements below is followed by five suggested answers or completions. Select the ONE that is best in each case.

1. A 35-year-old man presented to his physician complaining of morning headaches which had progressively worsened over the past 2 months. A magnetic resonance image (MRI) scan of his brain (shown in Figure 8.1) revealed a mass lesion suggestive of a primary brain tumor. All of the following are true about intracranial gliomas EXCEPT
    A. they are the most common intracranial tumor
    B. they rarely undergo malignant degeneration
    C. they almost never metastasize to other organs
    D. permanent cure is unlikely
    E. they typically arise in the cerebral hemispheres in adults

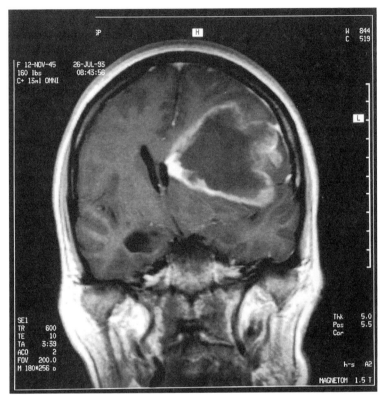

Figure 8.1

2. A 17-year-old female was admitted to the surgical intensive care
   unit for multiple traumatic injuries following a motor vehicle accident. She also sustained a severe closed head injury in addition
   to her other injuries. A MRI of the brain revealed multiple punctate hemorrhages, diffuse cerebral edema, and partially effaced
   basal cisterns. An intracranial pressure monitor was placed to
   monitor the patient's suspected intracranial hypertension. Intracranial pressure above what value requires treatment?

   A. 10 mm Hg
   B. 20 mm Hg
   C. 30 mm Hg
   D. 40 mm Hg
   E. 50 mm Hg

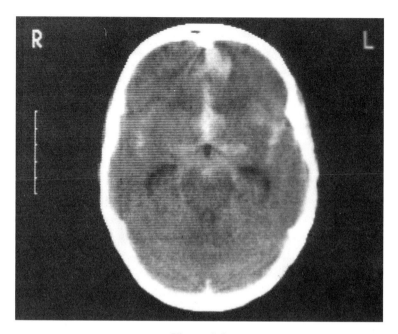

Figure 8.2

3. A 53-year-old man with no significant medical history presented to the emergency center with complaints of cataclysmic headache while engaging in sexual intercourse. This was accompanied by nausea, vomiting, nuchal rigidity with meningismus, and diffuse occipital headache. A CT scan (shown in Figure 8.2) confirmed subarachnoid hemorrhage. All of the following are true about subarachnoid hemorrhage EXCEPT
   A. it rarely occurs in sleep
   B. it can be precipitated by physical activity
   C. patients are frequently hypertensive following hemorrhage
   D. it causes retinal hemorrhages
   E. it causes changes in the electrocardiogram (ECG)

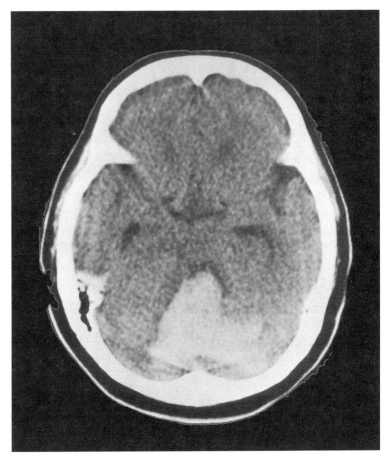

Figure 8.3

4. A 68-year-old male with a known history of hypertension and no
   other significant medical history presented complaining of a "stiff
   neck" associated with severe occipital headache. When he attempted to ambulate, he was markedly "dizzy" and uncoordi-
   nated, and he had associated vomiting. The computed tomography (CT) image of his head is shown in Figure 8.3. He is MOST
   likely to have had a
   A. seizure focus originating in the basal ganglia
   B. thalamic hemorrhage

C. pontine infarction
D. intracerebellar hemorrhage
E. frontal lobe infarction

5. Raised intracranial pressure can be treated with all of the following EXCEPT
   A. elevation of the head of the bed
   B. drainage of cerebrospinal fluid through a ventriculostomy
   C. hypoventilation
   D. intravenous mannitol
   E. intravenous urea

6. A growing skull fracture occurs
   A. only in children
   B. only over the parietal bone
   C. only along the base of the skull
   D. without a tear of the dura mater
   E. in adults with elevated intracranial pressure

7. A patient with mydriasis of the left pupil, right-sided hemiparesis, and an upgoing right plantar reflex is MOST likely to have herniation of the
   A. frontal lobe
   B. uncus
   C. diencephalon
   D. cerebellum
   E. visual cortex

8. A 45-year-old male presented to his family physician with complaints of occipital headache, hoarseness, difficulty swallowing, and ataxia. A MRI of the brain revealed the findings shown in Figures 8.4A and 8.4B. The patient's symptoms and MRI findings are MOST likely consistent with
   A. hydrocephalus
   B. stroke
   C. arteriovenous malformation (AVM)
   D. aneurysm
   E. choroid plexus papilloma

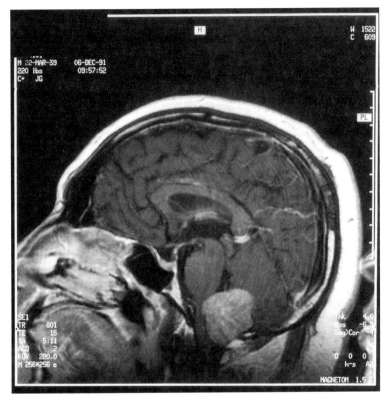

Figure 8.4A

9. A 63-year-old female presented with a left lower quadrant abdominal mass and distressing abdominal pain. She was discovered to have advanced left ovarian carcinoma, and she elected to have terminal care only. Her intractable left-sided abdominal pain is MOST likely to respond to
   A. dorsal root entry zone (DREZ) rhizotomy
   B. sympathectomy
   C. hemicordotomy
   D. cingulotomy
   E. pituitary ablation

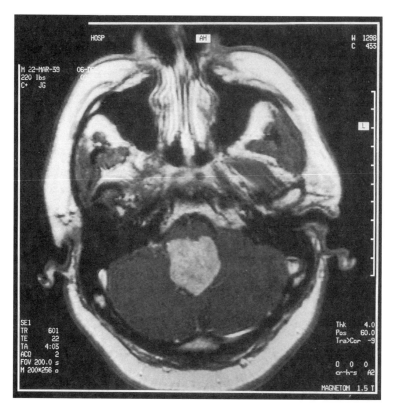

Figure 8.4B

10. The BEST surgical treatment for bone pain from widely metastatic breast or prostate cancer is
    A. DREZ rhizotomy
    B. sympathectomy
    C. cordotomy
    D. cingulotomy
    E. pituitary ablation

11. Patients with causalgia typically have all of the following EX-CEPT
   A. constant burning pain
   B. autonomic and trophic changes
   C. complete paralysis of the affected extremity
   D. a good response to sympathectomy
   E. pain worsened by rubbing or touching the affected extremity

---

DIRECTIONS (Questions 12 through 14): For each numbered word, phrase, or statement, select the ONE lettered heading that is most closely associated with it. Each lettered heading may be used once, more than once, or not at all.

   A. visual evoked potential
   B. brainstem auditory evoked potential
   C. somatosensory evoked potential
   D. nerve conduction velocity

12. Brachial plexus injury

13. Multiple sclerosis

14. Peripheral nerve entrapment

DIRECTIONS (Questions 15 through 22): Each of the questions or incomplete statements below is followed by five suggested answers or completions. Select the ONE that is best in each case.

---

15. All of the following characterize, or are associated with, a symptomatic herniated cervical disc EXCEPT
   A. hypesthesia, weakness, and reduction of deep tendon reflex
   B. interscapular pain
   C. pain often relieved by extension
   D. removal by anterior surgical approach
   E. lightning-like paresthesias extending to the limbs (Lhermitte's phenomenon)

16. Which of the following neurogenic tumors is NOT a glioma?
    A. ependymoblastoma
    B. neurinoma
    C. oligodendroglioma
    D. spongioblastoma
    E. medulloblastoma

17. If an otherwise well, middle-aged patient develops epilepsy, the presumptive diagnosis should be
    A. idiopathic
    B. arteriosclerosis
    C. cerebral tumor
    D. Parkinson's disease
    E. previous brain injury

18. Cerebrospinal fluid otorrhea is MOST often a result of
    A. fracture of the petrous ridge
    B. rupture of the tympanic membrane
    C. fracture of the cribriform plate
    D. fracture of the mastoid air cells
    E. fracture of the parietal bone

19. The estimated mean rate of axonal regeneration after peripheral nerve injury is
    A. 1 mm/day
    B. 1 mm/week
    C. 1 cm/week
    D. 10 cm/month
    E. 3 mm/week

20. The MOST malignant brain tumor is
    A. glioblastoma multiforme
    B. astrocytoma
    C. oligodendroglioma
    D. spongioblastoma
    E. ependymoma

21. Congenital malformations of the nervous system that are frequently associated with infantile hydrocephalus include all of the following EXCEPT
   A. Chiari II malformation
   B. meningoceles
   C. myelomeningoceles
   D. Dandy–Walker syndrome
   E. aqueductal stenosis

22. A 20-year-old male fell off his motorcycle and was found unconscious. When seen in the emergency room he was mentally clear, but over the next two hours he became confused, less responsive, and developed right-sided weakness. His CT scan (shown in Figure 8.5) reveals
   A. epidural hematoma
   B. subdural hematoma
   C. subarachnoid hematoma
   D. intraventricular hemorrhage
   E. intracerebral hemorrhage

Figure 8.5

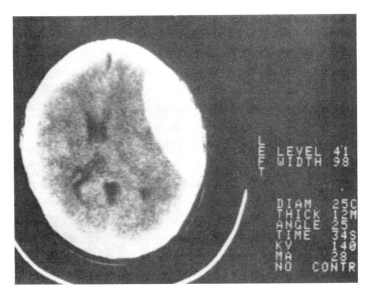

DIRECTIONS (Questions 23 through 26): For each numbered word, phrase, or statement select the ONE lettered heading that is most closely associated with it. Each lettered heading may be used once, more than once, or not at all.

A. meningocele
B. myelocele
C. encephalocele
D. syringomyelia

23. A pocket of fluid trapped within the spinal cord parenchyma

24. A membranous inclusion of cerebrospinal fluid

25. A protrusion of spinal cord and/or spinal nerves within the meningeal sac

26. Brain parenchyma protruding through a defect in the skull

DIRECTIONS (Questions 27 and 28): Each of the questions or incomplete statements below is followed by five suggested answers or completions. Select the ONE that is best in each case.

27. Which of the following is more descriptive of brain tumors in children than those in adults?
A. frequently supratentorial
B. frequently infratentorial
C. rarely produce hydrocephalus
D. usually occur near the gray/white junction
E. high-grade cerebellar astrocytoma

28. All of the following statements regarding extradural spinal tumors are true EXCEPT
A. they may produce paraplegia
B. they may produce pain
C. they are frequently malignant
D. they are frequently metastatic
E. they frequently arise from regional neural elements

Neurosurgery

Answers and Comments

1. **(B)** Recurrent gliomas often degenerate into more malignant variants, including glioblastoma. Note the cystic feature and mass effect that is characteristic of glioblastoma. (**Ref. 1,** p. 1244)

2. **(B)** Although intracranial pressure above 10 mm Hg is only infrequently noted in normal persons, pressure above 20 mm Hg is considered pathologic and requires treatment. (**Ref. 1,** p. 1253; **Ref. 2,** pp. 1834–1835)

3. **(A)** At least one-third of patients sustaining subarachnoid hemorrhage develop it during sleep. Note the hyperdense blood in the interhemispheric fissure, Sylvian fissures, and paramesencephalic cistern. This picture is characteristic of subarachnoid hemorrhage. (**Ref. 1,** p. 1246; **Ref. 2,** p. 1847)

4. **(D)** While headache and vomiting occur with hemorrhage in many locations, the combination of dizziness and ataxia is characteristic of cerebellar hemorrhages. Note the hyperdense blood in the posterior fossa. (**Ref. 1,** p. 1249; **Ref. 2,** p. 1850)

5. **(C)** Hypoventilation should be avoided because it contributes to increased intracranial pressure by increasing Pco_2, cerebral vasodilation, and ultimately cerebral blood flow. (**Ref. 1,** p. 282; **Ref. 2,** p. 1832)

6. **(A)** Growing skull fractures occur only in the presence of a growing, expandable child's skull. (**Ref. 1,** p. 1255)

7. **(B)** Uncal herniation compresses the ipsilateral third nerve and the parasympathetic pupilloconstrictor fibers in the periphery of the nerve, resulting in unopposed sympathetic input causing pupillary dilation. Motor fibers going to the contralateral extremities are compressed in the ipsilateral cerebral peduncle, thereby causing hemiparesis or hemiplegia. (**Ref. 1,** p. 1254)

8. **(E)** Although choroid plexus papillomas can cause hydrocephalus by oversecretion of spinal fluid, they may also cause focal compression of normal cerebrospinal fluid (CSF) drainage pathways. This particular patient does not show hydrocephalus, as the lateral, third, and fourth ventricles are normal in size, despite the choroid plexus papilloma of the fourth ventricle. Note the contrast enhancing mass that appears to be arising from the floor of the fourth ventricle. (**Ref. 1,** pp. 1271–1272)

9. **(C)** Contralateral hemicordotomy (sectioning of the spinothalamic tract) is most effective for unilateral pain from cancer. (**Ref. 1,** p. 1278; **Ref. 2,** pp. 1858–1859)

10. **(E)** Pituitary ablation, possibly by interrupting growth hormone stimulation of these tumors, results in decreased tumor size and amelioration of pain. (**Ref. 1,** p. 1280)

11. **(C)** Causalgia may occur after partial nerve injury. All findings listed are typical except complete paralysis. (**Ref. 1,** p. 1268; **Ref. 2,** p. 1859)

12. **(C)** Brachial plexus injuries frequently affect somatosensory signal transmission. (**Ref. 3,** p. 1847)

13. **(A)** Patients with multiple sclerosis may have optic neuritis, which slows conduction of visual evoked potentials. (**Ref. 3,** p. 816)

14. **(D)** Slowing of nerve conduction velocity is characteristic of peripheral nerve entrapment. (**Ref. 1,** p. 1268)

15. **(C)** Extension narrows the neural foramenae and often *increases* pain where degenerative facet joints and/or osteophytic spurs encroach upon the exiting nerve root. Both cervical and lumbar discs can compress nerve roots, resulting in decreased strength, sensation, and reflex activity. Interscapular pain may occur with lower cervical disc herniation. Herniated cervical discs are removed by either anterior or posterior surgical approaches (most commonly anterior). Lumbar discs are almost always removed by posterior approaches. Lhermitte's phenomenon, a lightning-like paresthesia extending down the spine and occasionally to the extremities, may occur with neck movement (especially extension) in patients with herniated cervical discs. (**Ref. 1,** pp. 1262, 1265, 1266; **Ref. 2,** pp. 1851–1852)

16. **(B)** Neurinomas are usually extracerebral tumors that arise from the nerve sheath. Within the cranial cavity, they usually arise from the eighth cranial nerve. All other tumors listed are types of gliomas. (**Ref. 1,** p. 1245)

17. **(C)** The onset of epilepsy in middle-aged patients should always raise the suspicion of a cerebral tumor, and it should be the presumptive diagnosis until definitively excluded. (**Ref. 2,** p. 1839)

18. **(A)** Cerebrospinal fluid (CSF) otorrhea is usually due to a fracture that involves the petrous part of the temporal bone with a tear into the subarachnoid space. This may cause liberation of CSF through the external auditory canal. (**Ref. 1,** p. 1190; **Ref. 2,** p. 1834)

19. **(A)** The mean rate of axonal regeneration following peripheral nerve injury is 1 mm/day. (**Ref. 1,** p. 1268; **Ref. 2,** p. 1839)

20. **(A)** Glioblastoma multiforme is the most malignant brain tumor and, unfortunately, the most frequent type of glioma. (**Ref. 1,** p. 1241)

21. **(B)** Pure meningoceles do not produce infantile hydrocephalus. The other conditions mentioned are usually associated with infantile hydrocephalus. (**Ref. 1,** pp. 1271–1272; **Ref. 2,** p. 1857)

22. **(A)** This history is classic for an epidural hematoma. The "lucid interval" is a feature of such, and the CT scan confirms the diagnosis. Most epidural hematomas are arterial in origin, but they can also arise from torn meningeal veins or venous sinuses. (**Ref. 1,** p. 1256; **Ref. 2,** p. 1835)

23. **(D)** Syringomyelia is an abnormal collection of fluid within the spinal cord parenchyma and may result from trauma, tumor, or congenital malformation. (**Ref. 1,** p. 1273; **Ref. 2,** p. 1875)

24. **(A)** A meningocele is a collection of fluid covered by meninges. (**Ref. 1,** p. 1270; **Ref. 2,** p. 1874)

25. **(B)** A myelocele, or truly a meningomyelocele, is a membranous sac into which the spinal cord and/or spinal nerves may protrude. (**Ref. 1,** p. 1270; **Ref. 2,** p. 1874)

26. **(C)** Encephalocele is a condition in which there is a protrusion of brain tissue, within the meningeal sac, through a defect in the skull. (**Ref. 1,** p. 1270)

27. **(B)** Approximately 70% of brain tumors in adults are supratentorial (eg, glioma, meningioma, pituitary adenomas, craniopharyngioma, dermoid, epidermoid, and lymphoma). Approximately 70% of brain tumors in children are infratentorial (eg, cerebellar astrocytoma, ependymoma, and medulloblastoma). Brain tumors in children are usually midline and infratentorial; consequently, they may produce hydrocephalus by direct pressure on the aqueduct and/or ventricular system. Cerebellar astrocytomas in children are usually low-grade and have a relatively good prognosis. (**Ref. 1,** pp. 1241–1242, 1244; **Ref. 2,** p. 1839)

28. **(E)** Spinal tumors are often distinguished as *extra*dural or *intra*dural. Most extradural spinal tumors are metastatic and malignant. Both extradural and intradural spinal tumors produce paraplegia and pain. Intradural spinal tumors are usually benign (meningiomas, neurofibromas, or schwannomas) and develop from local neural elements. (**Ref. 1,** pp. 1259–1261; **Ref. 2,** pp. 1844–1845)

9

Surgery of Trauma and Burns

Tina L. Palmieri
Michael H. Metzler

DIRECTIONS (Questions 1 through 43): Each of the questions or incomplete statements below is followed by five suggested answers or completions. Select the ONE that is best in each case.

1. The initial maneuver to establish an airway in a patient with multiple injuries is
   - **A.** oropharyngeal airway
   - **B.** uncuffed endotracheal tube
   - **C.** suctioning foreign debris and lifting up the mandible (jaw lift)
   - **D.** cuffed endotracheal tube
   - **E.** tracheostomy

2. Initial fluid resuscitation of a patient with multiple fractures and hypovolemic shock should be
   - **A.** blood transfusion
   - **B.** hypertonic saline
   - **C.** fresh frozen plasma

    D. Ringer's lactate
    E. albumin

3. What is the accuracy of peritoneal lavage in determining that intraperitoneal injury has occurred in blunt trauma patients?
    A. 15%
    B. 30%
    C. 50%
    D. 70%
    E. more than 85%

4. Which of the following is the MOST common site of deceleration injury to the thoracic aorta?
    A. at its origin
    B. after the origin of the innominate artery
    C. at the junction of the thoracic and abdominal aortas
    D. just distal to the ligamentum arteriosum
    E. between the common carotid and subclavian arteries

5. All of the following are useful methods of local treatment for snakebite EXCEPT
    A. immobilization
    B. venous tourniquet
    C. incision and suction
    D. excision
    E. cryotherapy

6. Improperly managed penetrating neck wounds may cause significant morbidity and mortality because of all of the following EXCEPT
    A. the neck has many vital structures in close proximity
    B. delayed hemorrhage may cause exsanguination
    C. the neck has poor blood supply, and infections are frequent
    D. unrecognized esophageal injury may lead to mediastinitis
    E. delayed hemorrhage may cause acute loss of airway

7. A 22-year-old man is admitted after an automobile accident. His respiratory rate is 25/min with complaint of left chest pain. Blood pressure is 120/95; pulse, 110. Chest x-ray shows left hemothorax, occupying 20% of the pleural space, and rib fractures. Immediate treatment is
   A. tube thoracostomy, left
   B. intercostal block and strapping
   C. bilateral tube thoracostomy
   D. pericardiocentesis
   E. endotracheal intubation, mechanical ventilation, and pleural aspiration

8. A victim is brought into the emergency room in shock, having sustained a single stab wound in the left anterior fifth intercostal space. The chest x-ray is shown in Figure 9.1. The injury shown is associated with all of the following EXCEPT
   A. distended neck veins
   B. muffled heart sounds
   C. widened (increased) pulse pressure
   D. hypotension
   E. shock

9. Select the appropriate order of priorities in the management of a patient with multiple injuries.
   1. splinting of fractures
   2. control of external hemorrhage
   3. relief of tension pneumothorax
   4. IV fluid treatment of shock
   5. maintenance of airway
   A. 4,5,3,1,2
   B. 5,4,1,2,3
   C. 5,3,2,4,1
   D. 3,2,1,4,5
   E. 2,4,3,5,1

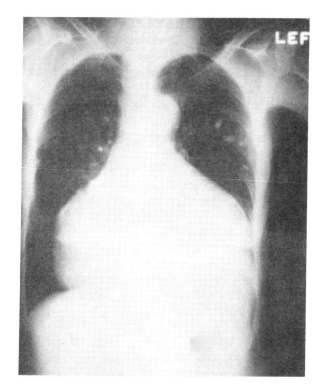

Figure 9.1

10. The major source of protein for multitrauma patients during the catabolic phase is
    A. plasma proteins
    B. fat
    C. liver
    D. skeletal muscle
    E. kidney

11. A patient with neck pain after a motor vehicle accident becomes tachypneic, tachycardic, and cyanotic. Oxygen saturation drops to 88% on 100% face mask. He is breathing spontaneously; breath sounds are equal bilaterally. What is the airway of choice?
 A. bag-mask ventilation
 B. orotracheal intubation
 C. nasotracheal intubation
 D. cricothyroidotomy
 E. tracheostomy

12. Which of the following findings suggests that shock in an injured patient may have a cause other than hypovolemia?
 A. hypotension
 B. distended neck veins
 C. decreased skin temperature
 D. diminished pulse pressure
 E. falling central venous pressure

13. The MOST common finding in patients surviving traumatic thoracic aortic injury from deceleration is
 A. respiratory distress
 B. widened or indistinct mediastinum on chest x-ray
 C. shock
 D. hoarseness
 E. shoulder pain

14. All of the following are physical signs of both massive hemothorax and tension pneumothorax EXCEPT
 A. tracheal shift
 B. decreased breath sounds
 C. tachycardia
 D. hypotension
 E. distended neck veins

15. A 20-year-old man falls from the roof of a two-story house, landing on a pile of rubble. The initial evaluation reveals an obvious flail chest with no other apparent injuries. The patient is in severe respiratory distress, breath sounds on the right are slightly decreased, and the percussion note is similar bilaterally, trachea midline. Arterial blood gases (with patient on facemask oxygen)

are: Pao_2, 45 mm Hg; $Paco_2$, 28 mm Hg; and pH, 7.47. What is the component of his injury that is MOST likely responsible for the abnormalities in his blood gases?
   A.   chest wall instability
   B.   pain
   C.   pulmonary contusion
   D.   hypovolemia
   E.   pneumothorax

16. Which of the following tests is MOST accurate in diagnosing suspected pancreatic injury?
   A.   elevated serum amylase
   B.   computed tomography (CT) scan of the abdomen
   C.   elevated white blood count (WBC)
   D.   high urine amylase
   E.   high serum lipase

17. A patient has been stabbed in the anterior abdomen. He has no intra-abdominal symptoms or signs. What is the MOST reliable diagnostic maneuver to rule out intra-abdominal injury?
   A.   peritoneal lavage
   B.   CT of the abdomen with contrast
   C.   CT of the abdomen without contrast
   D.   wound exploration
   E.   catheter contrast injection of the wound

18. What is the MOST common infecting organism in overwhelming postsplenectomy infection?
   A.   *Escherichia coli*
   B.   meningococcus
   C.   streptococcus
   D.   pneumococcus
   E.   staphylococcus

19. All of the following findings are characteristic of overwhelming postsplenectomy sepsis EXCEPT
   A.   shock
   B.   hyperglycemia
   C.   disseminated intravascular coagulation
   D.   sudden onset of symptoms
   E.   headache

20. For which of the following organ injuries is diagnostic peritoneal lavage (DPL) LEAST likely to be helpful?
    A. pancreas
    B. small intestine
    C. spleen
    D. sigmoid colon
    E. liver

21. Decreased $Paco_2$ levels should be attained in a patient at serious risk for cerebral edema secondary to a head injury in order to
    A. prevent neurogenic pulmonary edema
    B. allow reciprocally high levels of Pao_2 in the brain
    C. prevent increased capillary permeability
    D. prevent cerebral vasodilatation
    E. prevent metabolic acidosis

22. Brain injury alone
    A. frequently causes shock
    B. causes shock that is reversed by very simple measures
    C. causes shock only if the skull is intact
    D. rarely causes shock
    E. causes shock if hypoxia is superimposed

23. The level of consciousness for a head injury patient is BEST evaluated by
    A. Glasgow Coma Scale
    B. response to pain
    C. CT scan
    D. pupillary responses
    E. visual evoked potentials

24. The term "sacral sparing"
    A. refers to a fracture of the sacrum
    B. occurs with complete transection of the lumbosacral spinal cord
    C. is considered a diagnostic sign of spinal cord transection
    D. is considered a good prognostic sign in the presence of spinal cord injury
    E. is part of the spinal shock syndrome

25. A patient with severe hypovolemic shock will have all of the following EXCEPT
  A. loss of more than 40% of blood volume
  B. base excess
  C. low urinary output
  D. low blood pressure
  E. cool, pale extremities

26. All of the following findings suggest urethral injury EXCEPT
  A. blood at the external urethral meatus
  B. scrotal hematoma
  C. absence of a palpable prostate on rectal examination
  D. high-riding prostate on rectal examination
  E. blood in the rectal lumen

27. Rabies is seldom, if ever, a risk in bites from
  A. squirrels
  B. bats
  C. dogs
  D. cats
  E. raccoons

28. All of the following are appropriate treatments of extremity frostbite EXCEPT
  A. delayed warming if refreezing is possible
  B. water immersion at 40°C
  C. rapid rewarming
  D. vigorous massage
  E. allowing rewarming at room temperature

29. Which of the following is NOT commonly present in hypothermia at or below 32°C?
  A. mental aberration
  B. shivering
  C. hypokalemia
  D. hypotension and bradycardia
  E. gray, cyanotic skin

30. Regardless of the tetanus immunization status of a patient with a tetanus-prone wound, which of the following is mandatory?
    A. diphtheria, pertussis, and tetanus (DPT) toxoid injection
    B. diphtheria and tetanus (DT) toxoid injection
    C. tetanus immune globulin injection
    D. antibiotic coverage of tetanus organisms
    E. wound cleansing and debridement

31. All of the following are signs of acute vascular compromise of an extremity EXCEPT
    A. diminished sensation
    B. pallor
    C. absent pulses
    D. gangrene
    E. pain

32. In cases of pancreatic injury, the finding listed below which indicates the MOST serious pancreatic injury is
    A. serum amylase >250 units
    B. major pancreatic duct injury
    C. contusion with major duct intact
    D. serum calcium <8 mg/dL
    E. hyperglycemia

33. A gallbladder ruptured secondary to blunt abdominal trauma should be treated by
    A. serial CT and physical examinations
    B. placement of a T-tube in the common duct, regardless of other treatment
    C. cholecystectomy
    D. cholecystostomy
    E. Roux-en-Y cholecystojejunostomy

34. Which is the MOST commonly injured intra-abdominal organ in blunt trauma?
    A. liver
    B. kidney
    C. spleen
    D. stomach
    E. colon

35. Appropriate management of a .22-caliber gunshot wound traversing the neck may include all of the following EXCEPT
   A. observation only
   B. endotracheal intubation
   C. arteriography
   D. esophagoscopy
   E. bronchoscopy

36. The BEST diagnostic test for a bronchial transection is
   A. output from chest tubes
   B. bronchoscopy
   C. CT scanning
   D. plain tomography
   E. plain chest x-ray

37. True statements associated with burns include all of the following EXCEPT
   A. cardiac output initially falls in proportion to the area of the burn
   B. mortality is increased when accompanied by inhalation injury
   C. mortality expected from a 50% body surface area (BSA) burn is the same regardless of patient age
   D. pulmonary vascular resistance increases in the immediate postburn period
   E. the cellular immune response is depressed after burn injury

38. Regarding electrical injury, all of the following statements are true EXCEPT
   A. hyperkalemia may result from tissue necrosis
   B. myoglobin and hemoglobin pigment may produce renal failure
   C. heat is the principle mediator of tissue damage in high-voltage injuries
   D. heat production is related to tissue resistance
   E. the cutaneous lesion is frequently an accurate indicator of the extent of deep tissue injury

39. The preferred method of obtaining airway control in a 25-year-old unconscious, apneic patient with severe maxillofacial trauma is
   A. cricothyroidotomy
   B. nasotracheal intubation
   C. orotracheal intubation
   D. bag–mask ventilation
   E. facemask oxygen

40. Criteria for identification of injured patients who should be cared for in trauma centers, as opposed to in the nearest hospital, include all of the following EXCEPT
   A. physiologic or neurologic instability
   B. certain types of trauma requiring a system approach for care
   C. certain mechanisms of injury
   D. indigent patients with no insurance, regardless of degree of injury
   E. preexisting health conditions or extremes of age which will complicate care of the injuries

41. All of the following are common findings in the first 24 hours after inhalation injury with burn EXCEPT
   A. history of burn in an enclosed space
   B. hoarseness
   C. abnormal chest x-ray
   D. carbonaceous sputum
   E. bronchorrhea

42. Which of the following should NOT be used to control the pain caused by fractured ribs?
   A. morphine IV
   B. Demerol IM
   C. intercostal nerve blocks
   D. rib belts
   E. muscle relaxants

43. Clinical signs of burn wound infection include all of the following EXCEPT
   A. unexpectedly rapid eschar separation
   B. violaceous edematous wound margin

C. conversion of partial-thickness burn areas to full-thickness tissue necrosis
D. prolonged time to burn eschar separation
E. dark brown or black wound discoloration

DIRECTIONS (Questions 44 through 55): Each group of questions below consists of lettered headings followed by a list of numbered words, phrases, or statements. For each numbered word, phrase, or statement, select the ONE lettered heading that is most closely associated with it. Each lettered heading may be used once, more than once, or not at all.

Questions 44 through 50

A. DPL
B. CT scan
C. serial physical examinations
D. arteriogram
E. retrograde cystourethrogram

44. Useful in assessing retroperitoneal structures

45. Preferred test for evaluating potential abdominal solid organ injury

46. Preferred management of awake, alert trauma patient with mild abdominal tenderness being admitted for observation following a motor vehicle accident

47. Very sensitive diagnostic test for intraperitoneal injury, but not specific as to organ(s) injured

48. Indicated for evaluation of patient with blood at urethral meatus

49. Useful in identifying vascular injury after penetrating or blunt trauma

50. Useful in cases of penetrating neck trauma

Questions 51 through 55

    A. >100,000 RBC/mL
    B. clinical signs of peritoneal irritation
    C. chest tube placement
    D. hypotension in comatose multitrauma patient
    E. needle thoracentesis

51. Indication for DPL

52. Indication of positive DPL results in blunt trauma patient

53. Contraindication to peritoneal lavage

54. Immediate treatment of tension pneumothorax

55. Indicated for treatment of 40% pneumothorax following stab wound of the chest

---

DIRECTIONS (Questions 56 through 62): This section consists of a clinical situation followed by a series of questions. Study the situation and select the ONE best answer to each question following it.

A 25-year-old man weighing 70 kg was trapped in a house fire in which he sustained full-thickness burns to his entire head, neck, anterior trunk, and right arm, including the hand. On arrival he is confused. His respiratory rate is 25; BP, 170/90; and heart rate, 120 on 2 L nasal cannula with oxygen saturation of 100%. His eyebrows, eyelashes, and nasal hair are singed, and he is hoarse, with audible stridor. His burned areas are shown in Figure 9.2A.

56. What is the BEST method of initial airway management for this patient?
    A. continue with 2 L nasal cannula pending blood gas result
    B. 40% oxygen via face mask
    C. endotracheal intubation
    D. needle cricothyroidotomy
    E. tracheostomy

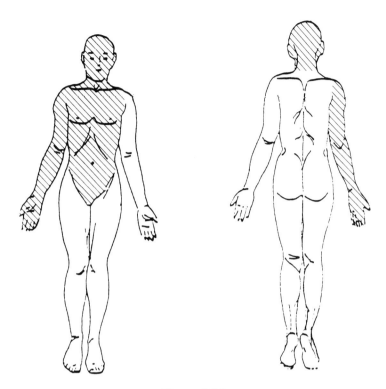

Figure 9.2A

57. The patient becomes increasingly combative. Appropriate initial
    treatment of the patient's agitation should include all of the fol-
    lowing EXCEPT
    A. administration of supplemental oxygen at 100%
    B. intravenous narcotics
    C. measurement of carboxyhemoglobin level
    D. assessment for associated head injury
    E. blood gas analysis

58. Using the "rule of nines," what percent of this patient's body is burned?

    A. 9
    B. 18
    C. 27
    D. 36
    E. 45

59. At what initial rate (using the Parkland formula) should intravenous lactated Ringer's solution be administered?

    A. 340 cc/hr
    B. 420 cc/hr
    C. 550 cc/hr
    D. 630 cc/hr
    E. 710 cc/hr

60. The patient's right upper extremity becomes cyanotic and cool, with delayed capillary refill, loss of pulses, and no flow signal on Doppler ultrasound exam. The nearest burn center is 3 hours away. Immediate treatment should include

    A. amputation
    B. escharotomy
    C. application of ice
    D. arteriogram
    E. intravenous heparin

61. As evaluation continues, the patient's blood pressure drops to 70/40, pulse is 170, and urine output is negligible. Appropriate initial management may include all of the following EXCEPT to

    A. increase rate of intravenous fluid administration
    B. administer lasix
    C. assess for occult blood loss
    D. check patency of Foley catheter
    E. institute central venous pressure monitoring

62. After appropriate intervention, blood pressure is 150/70, pulse is 120, and urine output is 40 cc/hr. Which of the following represent valid reasons for transfer to a burn unit?

    A.   presence of inhalation injury
    B.   facial burn
    C.   burn involving hands
    D.   extensive full-thickness burns
    E.   all of the above

Surgery of Trauma and Burns

Answers and Comments

1. **(C)** The upper airway of trauma patients often becomes obstructed either with debris or with the patients' soft tissues. The chin lift and jaw thrust maneuvers pull the tongue and oral musculature forward away from the pharynx, thus clearing the airway. Suctioning of debris also is helpful. If this not effective, endotracheal intubation may be indicated. (**Ref. 1,** p. 259)

2. **(D)** Ringer's lactate is the fluid of choice for initial resuscitation of patients with hypovolemic shock. Blood transfusion may not be necessary. Hypertonic saline will eventually result in excessive chloride and additional acidosis. Plasma and albumin have no improvement in outcome over Ringer's lactate. However, the cost of plasma and albumin is high, and there may be problems with hepatitis or increased pulmonary edema. (**Ref. 1,** p. 39)

3. **(E)** The accuracy of peritoneal lavage in determining the presence of intraperitoneal hemorrhage in diagnosis of abdominal trauma is more than 95%. DPL is considered to be the "gold standard" test for diagnosis of intraperitoneal injury. Unfortunately, it is incapable of discriminating between bleeding requiring surgery and that which does not. (**Ref. 1,** p. 266)

4. (D) The most common site of injury to the thoracic aorta is just distal to the ligamentum arteriosum. The descending aorta, which is fixed at the junction of the arch of the aorta with the descending aorta, becomes a focal point of rotational and deceleration forces. (**Ref. 1,** p. 264)

5. (E) Basic therapy for snakebite involves retarding absorption of venom, removing venom from the wound, neutralizing or reducing the effects of venom, and preventing complications. Cryotherapy is not useful in the management of snakebite and, in fact, may cause increased morbidity. (**Ref. 1,** pp. 250–251)

6. (C) The neck has a rich blood supply and is relatively resistant to infection. All of the other responses represent valid reasons for further evaluation of penetrating neck trauma. (**Ref. 1,** p. 284)

7. (A) Treatment of hemothorax, unless it is very minimal, is a tube thoracostomy. Intercostal block with strapping restricts chest wall movement and is contraindicated. (**Ref. 1,** p. 263)

8. (C) The chest x-ray shows a dilated cardiac shadow. In a patient with chest injury, this should raise a suspicion of cardiac tamponade. The pulse pressure (systolic BP–diastolic BP) decreases (or narrows) with cardiac tamponade. Beck's triad, consisting of distended neck veins, hypotension, and muffled heart sounds, is present in one-third of patients with cardiac tamponade. (**Ref. 1,** p. 263)

9. (C) The first order of priority in the management of a trauma patient with multiple injuries is airway maintenance. The second priority in this patient is the tension pneumothorax, since it is interfering with breathing and therefore adequate ventilation, as well as reducing venous return, resulting in shock. Once airway and ventilation have been secured, control of hemorrhage is the highest priority in order to reduce volume loss and necessity for replacement. The fluid management of shock follows external hemorrhage control. Any blood loss that is prevented is blood that will not need to be replaced. Therefore, shock follows hemorrhage. The correction of shock is extremely important, and correction should occur as quickly as possible. Splinting of fractures is the last priority among those listed. Often these treatments may be performed simultaneously by multiple personnel. (**Ref. 1,** p. 259)

10. **(D)** The stored protein source used by the body during the catabolic phase is generated from skeletal muscles. There is subsequent loss of muscle mass. (**Ref. 1,** p. 110)

11. **(C)** Nasotracheal intubation minimizes manipulation of the neck during intubation and establishes an effective cuffed airway. The neck should be immobilized with in-line stabilization during the procedure. Spontaneous respiratory effort is needed for this intubation technique. (**Ref. 1,** p. 259)

12. **(B)** Distended neck veins indicate increased venous pressure and therefore a more central cause of shock, such as cardiac tamponade or tension pneumothorax. (**Ref. 1,** p. 263)

13. **(B)** Thoracic aortic disruption has relatively few symptoms until free rupture and immediate death. An x-ray finding of a widened and/or indistinct mediastinal silhouette is the most common sign and should raise suspicion of such an injury. Only 20% to 43% of patients with a widened mediastinum will have aortic disruptions. (**Ref. 1,** p. 264)

14. **(E)** Because of blood loss, a patient with massive hemothorax may not have elevated venous pressure. In such a case, the neck veins will be flat. (**Ref.1,** pp. 262–263)

15. **(C)** The $Paco_2$ indicates that the patient is hyperventilating. The low Pao_2 suggests shunting compatible with pulmonary contusion. Although the patient most likely has some chest instability, this alone cannot account for the degree of shunting he displays. (**Ref. 1,** pp. 261–262)

16. **(B)** CT scan has a sensitivity and specificity of greater than 80%, while elevated serum amylase is present in only 60% of patients with pancreatic injury. (**Ref. 1,** p. 275)

17. **(D)** Direct wound exploration with visualization of the bottom of the knife tract excludes or confirms peritoneal penetration.

When performed correctly, there is a false-negative rate of 0%. (**Ref. 1,** p. 266)

18. **(D)** Pneumococcus in the infecting agent in over 50% of overwhelming postsplenectomy infections. Asplenic individuals have decreased phagocytic ability of alveolar macrophages as well as decreased antibody response to antigens, thus lowering immunity. (**Ref. 1,** p. 267)

19. **(B)** Postsplenectomy sepsis is characterized by severe hypoglycemia, shock, sudden onset of symptoms, headache, and DIC (disseminated intravascular coagulopathy). (**Ref. 1,** p. 267)

20. **(A)** Since the pancreas is retroperitoneal, lavage of the peritoneal cavity may not provide diagnostic results. Frequently, however, there are associated intraperitoneal organ injuries which would make DPL positive. (**Ref. 1,** p. 274)

21. **(D)** Arterial carbon dioxide concentration is the most potent known regulator of cerebral vessel size. Cerebral vasodilation will increase cerebral blood volume, with a resultant increase in intracranial pressure. For serious head injuries, hyperventilation to attain $Paco_2$ values in the mid-20s may be necessary. (**Ref. 1,** p. 282)

22. **(D)** If a patient has a serious brain injury and is in shock, the cause of treatable hypotension should be sought elsewhere. Increasing intracranial pressure normally increases blood pressure and reduces heart rate. Hypotension due solely to brain injury is usually due to completed brainstem herniation, which is not reversible. (**Ref. 1,** p. 282)

23. **(A)** The Glasgow Coma Scale is the best known method of evaluating and following the level of consciousness. The scale ranges from 3 to 15 and assesses neurologic status based on eye opening, best verbal response, and best motor response. (**Ref. 1,** pp. 260, 282)

24. **(D)** Sacral sparing of neurologic function suggests an incomplete spinal cord injury. Motor or sensory function may be intact

below the injury level with an incomplete spinal cord injury. Sensation in the perineum and lower voluntary sphincter contraction should always be tested. (**Ref. 1,** p. 283)

25. **(B)** Patients with severe hypovolemic shock are generally hypotensive and demonstrate evidence of adrenergic discharge. There is usually lactic acidosis present that erodes the normal buffer base producing a base deficit. All the other answers are typical physiologic responses to severe hypovolemia. (**Ref. 1,** p. 37)

26. **(E)** All of the findings suggest urethral injury except blood in the rectal lumen, which suggests injury to the anus, rectum, or colon. All other findings would require urethrogram before insertion of a Foley catheter. (**Ref. 1,** p. 280)

27. **(A)** Rabies is not endemic in rodents. Bites by rats, mice, chipmunks, squirrels, rabbits, or other rodents have never been proven to produce human rabies, and postexposure prophylaxis is currently not indicated. (**Ref. 1,** p. 251)

28. **(D)** In treating frostbite, all wet and constricting clothing should be removed and patients wrapped in warm blankets. Rapid rewarming is the most effective therapy. Warming should be delayed only if refreezing is possible. Massage or use of ice water will increase tissue damage. (**Ref. 1,** p. 205)

29. **(B)** Shivering is frequently absent in hypothermic patients, especially if heat loss has occurred slowly. The elderly are particularly susceptible to hypothermia due to decreased ability to both generate and preserve heat. (**Ref. 1,** p. 207)

30. **(E)** Regardless of the active immunization status of a patient, meticulous surgical care with removal of all devitalized tissue and foreign bodies should be provided for all wounds. (**Ref. 1,** p. 290)

31. **(D)** Vascular compromise of an extremity is characterized by pain, pallor, pulselessness, paresthesias, and paralysis. Gangrene is not found in the acute setting but develops later. (**Ref. 1,** p. 289)

32. **(B)** Major ductal injury is the most serious finding listed. Ninety percent of patients with pancreatic injury have at least one associated injury. The presence or absence of pancreatic ductal injury is the major determinant of long-term survival. (**Ref. 1,** p. 274)

33. **(C)** Rupture of the gallbladder from blunt trauma is best treated by cholecystectomy, which is also the treatment of choice for severe contusion, avulsion, or perforation of the gallbladder. (**Ref. 1,** p. 270)

34. **(C)** The spleen is the most frequently injured organ, followed by the liver. The liver is the most frequently injured intraperitoneal organ in penetrating trauma. (**Ref. 1,** p. 266)

35. **(A)** Because of the presence of multiple vital structures in the neck, penetrating wounds through the sternocleidomastoid muscle have high risk of injury to signficant blood vessels, airway, or esophagus. Fifty percent of deaths due to penetrating neck trauma are preventable. Observation alone is not indicated. (**Ref. 1,** pp. 284–285)

36. **(B)** Although bronchial disruption may be suggested by continued pneumothorax after chest tube placement, persistent pneumothorax, or via CT or plain tomography findings, the definitive diagnosis is established by bronchoscopy. (**Ref. 1,** p. 263)

37. **(C)** The mortality rate for similar percent body surface area burns varies with age and preexisting health conditions. Inhalation injury potentiates the lethality of burns. Both cardiac and immune system function are diminished in the immediate postburn period. (**Ref. 1,** pp. 180–183)

38. **(E)** Electrical current may injure deep structures and leave the overlying skin intact, minimizing the apparent injury. This may lead to underresuscitation and subsequent renal failure due to myoglobin release and deposition in the renal tubules. (**Ref. 1,** p. 195)

39. **(A)** Cricothyroidotomy should be used when rapid airway control is indicated and injuries preclude orotracheal or nasotracheal intubation. Bag–mask and facemask oxygen do not provide ade-

quate airway control. The neck should be immobilized during this procedure. (**Ref. 1,** p. 259)

40. **(D)** A patient's social or economic status should not enter into triage considerations. All other answers are indications for triage of a patient to a trauma center. (**Ref. 1,** p. 294)

41. **(C)** Chest x-ray is insensitive in the detection of inhalation injury, even when severe injury exists. Bronchoscopy should be performed after the patient is hemodynamically stable to confirm or exclude injury, as well as to remove debris. (**Ref. 1,** p. 188)

42. **(D)** Rib belts or constrictive taping should be avoided because the reduced chest motion increases the incidence of retained secretions and atelectasis. (**Ref. 1,** p. 261)

43. **(D)** Delayed burn eschar separation is rarely due to subeschar sepsis. All of the other listed findings are classic signs of burn wound infection. (**Ref. 1,** p. 199)

44. **(B)** CT scan is extremely useful in identifying retroperitoneal injuries, which cannot be adequately assessed by DPL. (**Ref. 1,** p. 266)

45. **(B)** CT offers good visualization of solid organs and is "less invasive" than arteriogram. (**Ref. 1,** p. 266)

46. **(C)** Repeated physical exam is the best method of complete diagnosis in the multitrauma patient. Often minor injuries are not appreciated on initial exam. Continued vigilance with serial exams will often disclose further injuries. (**Ref. 1,** p. 259)

47. **(A)** DPL is the mainstay for diagnosis of presence of intraperitoneal hemorrhage. However, it gives no information on the exact site of injury. (**Ref. 1,** p. 266)

48. **(E)** Blood at the urethral meatus is one indication of possible urethral injury. A urethrogram is indicated prior to attempted catheter passage. Blind catheter passage with a urethral injury may make the injury worse. (**Ref. 1,** p. 278)

49. (D) Arteriogram is the "gold standard" in defining arterial injury after trauma. (**Ref. 1,** pp. 289–290)

50. (D) Arteriography looking for specific vascular injury is frequently indicated in penetrating neck trauma. (**Ref. 1,** p. 285)

51. (D) DPL is indicated because physical exam to exclude intra-abdominal injury is unreliable in a comatose patient. (**Ref. 1,** p. 266)

52. (A) One of the positive criteria for DPL in a blunt trauma patient is >100,000 RBC/mL lavage fluid. Other criteria include >500 WBC/mL, presence of bile or particulate matter in lavage fluid. (**Ref. 1,** p. 266)

53. (B) DPL is not indicated in patients who have clinical indications for operation such as diffuse peritonitis, evisceration, and gunshot wound. Overall sensitivity of DPL is 95%, specificity 98%. (**Ref. 1,** p. 266)

54. (E) Needle thoracentesis is the preferred initial treatment for tension pneumothorax because it is more rapid than chest tube insertion. Patients with tension pneumothorax are frequently moribund. A chest tube is definitive therapy, but its insertion may take additional time. A chest tube should be placed after needle thoracentesis has been performed. (**Ref. 1,** p. 260)

55. (C) In this situation, needle thoracentesis is not indicated. Definitive therapy for a pneumothorax, consisting of chest tube insertion, should be performed. (**Ref. 1,** p. 261)

56. (C) Both the history and physical findings suggest that the patient has sustained a significant upper airway injury. Hoarseness and stridor indicate that supraglottic edema has already created a partial upper airway obstruction. Prompt endotracheal intubation is indicated to maintain a patent airway. (**Ref. 1,** p. 178)

57. (B) The burn patient with upper airway injury may be confused secondary to carbon monoxide toxicity, associated head trauma, hypovolemic shock, hypoxia, or hypercarbia. Carbon monoxide displaces oxygen from the hemoglobin molecule, thus reducing

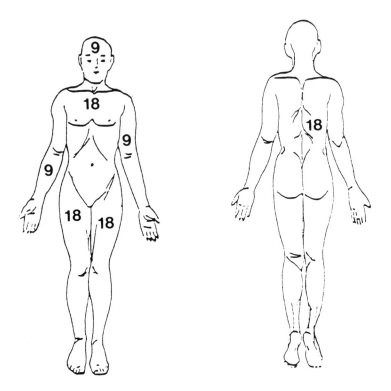

Figure 9.2B

its oxygen-carrying capacity. Treatment of carbon monoxide toxicity includes administration of 100% oxygen, which displaces carbon monoxide from the hemoglobin molecule. Narcotics and sedatives should be avoided until the cause of confusion is established. (**Ref. 1,** p. 178)

58. (D) The rule of nines is used to estimate the extent of body surface involvement. In an adult, each upper limb represents 9%; head and neck, 9%; each lower limb, 18%; anterior and posterior trunk, each 18%; perineum and genitalia, 1% (see Figure 9.2B). (**Ref. 1,** p. 179)

59. (D) The Parkland formula estimates fluid requirements for the first 24 hours postburn using the equation 4cc/kg/%BSA burn, which is 10,080 cc (4 × 70 × 36) in this case. Half of this volume (5040 cc) is administered in the first eight hours after injury, in this case at a rate of 630 cc/hour. This formula is merely an estimate of fluid needs; fluid rate is adjusted to maintain a urine output of 0.5 cc/kg/hr in adults. (**Ref. 1,** p. 185)

60. **(B)** Edema beneath an inelastic eschar may compromise blood flow to burned tissue. Escharotomy is indicated in full-thickness circumferential burns of extremities or thoracic wall when deterioration of peripheral circulation or ventilatory exchange, respectively, occurs. Figure 9.3 depicts an upper extremity escharotomy.

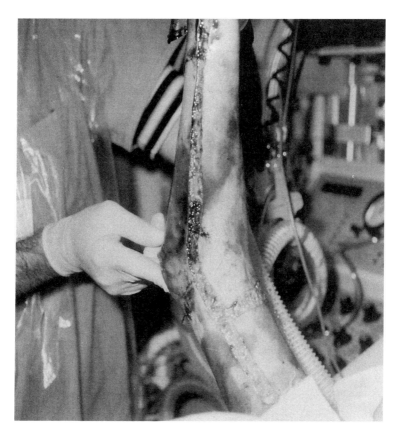

Figure 9.3

Direct application of ice is contraindicated in the treatment of burns. (**Ref. 1,** p. 178)

61. (**B**)   This patient is in hypovolemic shock due to volume depletion until proven otherwise and requires additional fluid administration. Lasix is contraindicated in the hypovolemic patient and will only exacerbate fluid abnormalities. (**Ref. 1,** p. 186)

62. (**E**)   All of the responses are appropriate reasons for transfer of a patient to a burn center for definitive care. Additional criteria for transfer include burn >10% in the elderly (>50 years old) or children (<10 years old); burns involving the perineum, hands, feet, or face; electrical or chemical injury; or patients with complicating medical problems. Direct contact with the burn center is imperative prior to transport. Wounds should be covered by a clean sheet for transfer. (**Ref. 1,** p. 178)

10

Orthopaedic Surgery
Barry J. Gainor
James M. Banovetz Jr.

DIRECTIONS (Questions 1 through 14): Each of the questions or incomplete statements below is followed by five suggested answers or completions. Select the ONE that is best in each case.

---

1. While treating a fracture in a cast
   A. it is unnecessary to immobilize the nearby joints
   B. occasionally the joints are immobilized
   C. immobilization of the joints leads to unnecessary joint fixation
   D. only the proximal joint is immobilized
   E. joints proximal and distal to the fracture should be immobilized

2. A 32-year-old woman is one day status-post long arm casting of her right arm for a Colles' fracture. Her arm is elevated, she has brisk capillary refill, and her fingers are not swollen. She does mention, however, that the pads of her thumb and index finger feel "numb and tingly." This finding is indicative of
   A. displacement of fragments
   B. excessive callus formation
   C. pressure on the median nerve
   D. pressure on the radial nerve
   E. pressure on the ulnar nerve

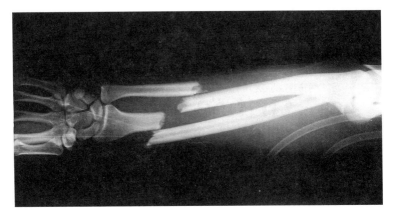

Figure 10.1

3. A 21-year-old man falls from a horse and sustains a fracture of both bones in the forearm in the midshaft region. His x-ray is shown in Figure 10.1. Physical examination reveals that neurovascular function of the hand is preserved. The MOST appropriate definitive treatment would include
   A. closed reduction and casting with end-to-end apposition of the fragments and minimal displacement
   B. closed reduction and casting with side-to-side ("bayonet") apposition of the fragments
   C. open reduction and plating of both bones to restore precise anatomic alignment
   D. splinting of the fracture without attempting a reduction
   E. open reduction to restore precise anatomic alignment followed by cast application

4. A 14-month-old female child presents to the emergency room with a history of fever to 104°F and unwillingness to walk. The child's past history has been unremarkable; she began ambulating at 11 months. Range of motion of her legs causes only minimal discomfort. The next and MOST important step in evaluating the patient for acute osteomyelitis is
   A. x-ray of the bone
   B. blood cultures
   C. x-ray of the adjoining joint

D. palpation for local bony tenderness
E. constitutional disturbances

5. A 47-year-old construction worker falls about 12 feet from a scaffold, landing on his feet and then his buttocks. He complains of severe left foot and lower back pain. On exam, he has a severely swollen left foot but is neurovascularly intact in both lower extremities. The MOST common foot fracture that occurs in this setting is
   A. medial malleolus
   B. talus
   C. lateral malleolus
   D. navicular
   E. calcaneus

6. A 95-year-old nursing home resident presents to the emergency room after being found on the floor next to her bed. She is unable to give a history but transfer records from an outside hospital indicate that she has a displaced hip fracture. They do not indicate which side, but this is clinically apparent because the affected limb is
   A. shortened
   B. externally rotated
   C. shortened and externally rotated
   D. flexed, abducted, and internally rotated
   E. flexed, abducted, and externally rotated

7. A 24-year-old man is involved in a motor vehicle accident and is referred to your facility with a diagnosis of a dislocated hip. If this is the MOST common type of dislocation, the involved limb will be in a position of
   A. flexion and adduction of hip
   B. extension of hip and knee
   C. flexion of hip and extension of knee
   D. neutral position
   E. external rotation of hip

8. A 12-year-old boy presents to your clinic with a complaint of pain and swelling of his right knee for about 1 month. This history, along with radiographic, magnetic resonance imaging (MRI), and tissue biopsy findings, is suggestive of osteogenic sarcoma. No evidence of metastasis is found. The family should be counseled that initial treatment for this disease must include

    A. radiotherapy

    B. chemotherapy

    C. curettage

    D. simple excision of the mass

    E. amputation or wide radical excision with reconstruction

9. An 18-year-old college student falls while mountain biking, landing on her outstretched left (nondominant) hand. She complains of wrist pain and is diffusely tender there. Neurovascular exam of her hand is unremarkable. You place her in a wrist splint because her MOST likely injury (one that is often not apparent on initial radiographs) is

    A. dislocated lunate

    B. fractured scaphoid

    C. retrolunar dislocation of capitate

    D. fractured lunate

    E. ligament tear

10. A 53-year-old farmer gets his arm caught in a power take-off and sustains an open fracture of his forearm bones. His hand neurovascular exam is intact, but the fractured end of his proximal radius fragment protrudes from a 6-cm wound on his dorsal forearm. He will require multiple trips to the operating room due to the MOST common complication of an open fracture, which is

    A. uncontrolled hemorrhage

    B. shortening

    C. infection

    D. comminution

    E. muscle contracture

11. A 45-year-old woman experiences severe back and left lower leg pain while making a bed. She has had recurrent episodes of mild localized back pain in the past, but no other significant past medical history. All of the following are suggestive of a herniated lumbar disk EXCEPT

A. incontinence of urine
B. weakness of great toe extension
C. diminished ankle jerk reflex
D. extensor plantar (Babinski) reflex
E. pain shooting down leg and into foot with straight leg raising

12. Clinical features of achondroplasia include all of the following EXCEPT

A. trident hand
B. mental deficiency
C. globular skull
D. dwarfism
E. prognathism

13. Pyogenic arthritis is common in all of the following EXCEPT

A. patients with debilitating disease
B. patients on cortisone therapy
C. rheumatoid arthritis
D. young people active in sports
E. premature infants

14. A 49-year-old immigrant from an underdeveloped country has a history suggestive of chronic active tuberculosis. He complains of diffuse pain in the locations listed below. Which area is most likely to demonstrate an osteoarticular tuberculous lesion on radiographic examination?

A. spine
B. hip
C. knee
D. shoulder
E. wrist

DIRECTIONS (Questions 15 through 18): The group of questions below consists of lettered headings followed by a list of numbered words, phrases, or statements. For each numbered word, phrase, or statement, select the ONE lettered heading that is most closely associated with it. Each lettered heading may be used once, more than once, or not at all.

    A. spondylosis
    B. spondylolysis
    C. spondylolisthesis
    D. spondylitis

15. Bony defect in the neural arch

16. Inflammation of the spine

17. Slipping of the body of one vertebra over the body of the next one below

18. Osteoarthritis of the spine in which hypertrophic spurs may impinge on nerve roots

DIRECTIONS (Questions 19 through 28): Each of the questions or incomplete statements below is followed by five suggested answers or completions. Select the ONE that is best in each case.

19. True statements concerning internal fixation of a fracture include all of the following EXCEPT
    A. it leads to increased damage to soft tissue
    B. it leads to increased damage to bone
    C. it is a potential source of infection in a wound
    D. it is essential in the treatment of all fractures
    E. it improves anatomic alignment of displaced fractures

20. Indications for total hip replacement include all of the following EXCEPT
    A. osteoarthritis
    B. osteonecrosis

C. rheumatoid arthritis
D. gonococcal arthritis
E. femoral neck fracture of an arthritic hip

21. A 36-year-old woman is an unrestrained passenger in a motor vehicle accident, sustaining the injury shown on the radiograph in Figure 10.2. She is neurovascularly intact in this extremity. Following successful reduction, the patient has considerable pain relief and remains neurovascularly intact. Prior to discharge, she should be counseled about the possibility of *late* complications, including all of the following EXCEPT
A. avascular necrosis of the femoral head
B. sciatic neuropathy
C. osteoarthritis
D. lengthening of the affected leg
E. decreased range of motion

Figure 10.2

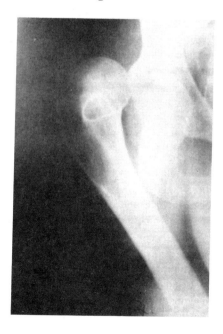

22. A 55-year-old woman with a long history of rheumatoid arthritis complains of pain and decreased motion of her right (dominant) wrist. She has marked swelling of her wrist, along with other rheumatoid deformities of her hand, but has good finger strength and range of motion. She is scheduled for dorsal wrist synovectomy because it will accomplish all of the following EXCEPT
    A. it requires joint replacement
    B. it effectively relieves pain
    C. it protects against tendon destruction
    D. it increases flexibility of the joint
    E. it removes diseased tissue

23. You are asked to see an infant in the newborn nursery regarding a possible developmental (congenital) dysplasia of the hip. All of the following physical exam signs are suggestive of this disorder in the newborn infant EXCEPT
    A. limitation of abduction
    B. a click with downward pressure on the flexed and abducted leg (Barlow's test)
    C. a click with upward pressure on the posterior aspect of the flexed and abducted leg (Ortolani's test)
    D. apparent shortening of the thigh or asymmetric skin folds
    E. pelvic tilt with standing on one leg (Trendelenburg's sign)

24. A 14-year-old girl is referred to you for follow-up of spondylolisthesis. Findings on her work-up may include all of the following EXCEPT
    A. a family history of the disorder and descendence from an inbred population
    B. nerve root as well as back pain
    C. normal "scottie dog" appearance of the posterior spinal elements on oblique radiographs
    D. 50% forward slip of the L5 vertebra on the S1 vertebra
    E. adequate relief of her symptoms with nonoperative treatment

25. Pathologic fractures occur with all of the following EXCEPT
    A. malignant tumors
    B. developmental diseases of bone
    C. metabolic conditions
    D. single-bone congenital abnormalities
    E. benign tumors

26. A 21-year-old college football player sustains a blow to the lateral aspect of his knee while his foot is planted. Lachman and pivot shift testing reveal a rupture of his anterior cruciate ligament. Varus/valgus stress testing reveal a commonly associated injury to the

    A. lateral collateral ligament
    B. popliteus muscle
    C. patellar ligament
    D. medial collateral ligament
    E. medial head of the gastrocnemius muscle

27. A 19-year-old man presents to the emergency room after a motor-cycle accident complaining of severe thigh pain. He has swelling and tenderness of the thigh, but distal neurovascular exam is intact. Radiographs reveal a comminuted and displaced fracture of the femur. Optimal treatment of this injury would be

    A. application of a traction boot and immobilization until the swelling subsides
    B. immediate internal fixation of the fracture
    C. application of a cylinder cast for six weeks
    D. insertion of a tibial traction pin with balanced traction to produce anatomic reduction and continued nonoperative management in this manner
    E. immediate placement of external fixator

28. A young woman falls on her arm, fracturing the humerus above the elbow. She has normal sensation in the palmar aspect of her hand, and she can spread her fingers and oppose her thumb normally. She cannot extend her hand at the wrist and has loss of sensation on the back of her hand. The structure injured, in addition to the humerus, is the

    A. median nerve
    B. ulnar nerve
    C. radial nerve
    D. musculocutaneous nerve
    E. brachial plexus

204 / Orthopaedic Surgery

DIRECTIONS (Questions 29 through 32): The group of questions below consists of lettered headings followed by a list of numbered words, phrases, or statements. For each numbered word, phrase, or statement, select the ONE lettered heading that is most closely associated with it. Each lettered heading may be used once, more than once, or not at all.

    A. may result in growth disturbance
    B. fatigue or stress fracture
    C. paralytic ileus
    D. fracture of the fibular shaft

29. Needs little or no formal fracture treatment

30. Associated with fracture of the thoracic or lumbar vertebra

31. Results from repetitive minor trauma

32. Fracture through the epiphyseal plate

DIRECTIONS (Questions 33 through 50): Each of the questions or incomplete statements below is followed by five suggested answers or completions. Select the ONE that is best in each case.

33. An 18-year-old man is struck by a car and sustains a closed fracture of the tibia and fibula with minimal displacement. A long-leg cast is applied, and the patient is admitted to the hospital. He is started on intravenous fluids and supplemental oxygen for fat emboli syndrome prophylaxis. Clinical signs MOST commonly associated with this syndrome are
    A. rising pulse and respiratory rate
    B. tachypnea and dyspnea
    C. petechiae over the chest
    D. confusion and delirium
    E. all of the above

34. A fracture through the pedicle of the axis (C2 vertebra) is known as
   A. Jefferson fracture
   B. hangman's fracture
   C. teardrop fracture
   D. fracture of Luschka
   E. none of the above

35. A patent is referred to your facility after a motor vehicle accident with a report of acute paralysis below the waist. The MOST dependable sign of a complete spinal cord injury is
   A. complete loss of temperature sensation and proprioception during the first 24 hours after injury
   B. complete loss of vibratory sensation and deep pain, especially in the extremities, during the first 4 hours after injury
   C. complete loss of motor and sensory function, including perianal sensation, 48 hours after injury
   D. loss of the bulbocavernosus reflex
   E. hyperreflexia

36. A 19-year-old rugby player is injured when a fellow player lands on his arm. He presents with his arm at his side, held by the opposite hand. A radiographic shoulder series, including anterior–posterior (AP), lateral scapular, and axillary views, reveal an anterior shoulder dislocation. In relating the circumstances of his injury, he will probably describe
   A. a severe traction injury on the extremity
   B. forceful internal rotation and traction
   C. forced abduction, extension, and external rotation of the extremity
   D. forward flexion of the shoulder with direct axial load
   E. none of the above

37. After reduction, the patient in the previous question reports numbness and tingling of his upper arm and demonstrates weakness in abduction. This common finding is the result of injury to the
    A. long thoracic nerve
    B. suprascapular nerve
    C. musculocutaneous nerve
    D. axillary nerve
    E. ulnar nerve

38. Which fractures require only symptomatic treatment?
    A. scapula and clavicle
    B. clavicle and humerus
    C. scapula and humerus
    D. humerus and fibula
    E. all of the above

39. An 8-year-old girl falls from the uneven bars during a gymnastics practice, sustaining a fracture of both bones of the forearm. The fractures are displaced and angulated. With considerable growth and remodelling potential remaining, the appropriate treatment for this injury is
    A. closed reduction and casting with end-to-end apposition of the fragments and minimal displacement
    B. closed reduction and casting with side-to-side ("bayonet") apposition of the fragments
    C. open reduction and plating of both bones to restore precise anatomic alignment
    D. splinting of the fracture without attempting a reduction
    E. open reduction to restore precise anatomic alignment followed by cast application

40. A 9-year-old girl falls from the uneven bars during a gymnastics practice and suffers a supracondylar fracture of her humerus. She has only a weak pulse by Doppler exam initially but is otherwise neurovascularly intact. After closed reduction and percutaneous pin fixation she is transferred to the floor. Close observation and rapid intervention are needed to avoid the serious complication of
    A. Volkmann's ischemic contracture
    B. nonunion of the healing fracture

C. a cubitus varus (gunstock deformity)
D. radial nerve palsy
E. median nerve palsy

41. A 3-year-old child falls while walking hand-in hand with his mother and presents with painful elbow. He is holding the elbow in full pronation and near full extension. Diagnosed with "pulled" or "nursemaid's" elbow, a reduction maneuver of supination and flexion results in a "click" sensation and relief of his symptoms. The injury involved was a
A. momentary dislocation of the humeral ulnar joint
B. hyperextension of the elbow
C. hyperpronation of the forearm
D. momentary dislocation of the radial capitellar joint
E. subluxation of the radial head through the annular ligament

42. You are consulted on an infant in the newborn nursery for a severe clubfoot deformity. You reassure the parents that, although she will require serial casts and probably a posteromedial release at about one year of age, she will eventually have near normal function of her foot. The components of the deformity that you describe to them are
A. equinus only
B. heel varus only
C. heel valgus and forefoot abductus
D. equinus, heel varus, and forefoot adductus
E. equinus, heel valgus, and metatarsus abductus

43. A 35-year-old do-it-yourselfer strikes his thumbnail with a hammer and presents with severe pain. Rapid relief should be provided by
A. alternating warm and cold soaks
B. immobilization with a splint and elevation
C. ice on the fingernail
D. warm soaks three times daily
E. decompression of the hematoma by making a hole in the fingernail

44. A 33-year-old woman was an unrestrained passenger in a motor vehicle accident and is brought to the emergency room in severe shock. Radiographs reveal a wide diastasis of her symphysis and a left iliac fracture. Rapid reduction and external fixation of her pelvis are necessary to treat the common, life-threatening complication of

    A. massive hemorrhage

    B. bladder injury

    C. rectal injury

    D. sciatic nerve injury

    E. leg shortening

45. A closed femur fracture may be the site of how many units of blood loss?

    A. up to one unit

    B. 2 to 3 units

    C. 4 units

    D. never more than 5 units

    E. 10 units

46. A 17-year-old man wrecks his off-road motorcycle, and the emergency personnel on the scene report that his right knee appears to be dislocated. On work-up in the emergency room, he has a swollen, tender knee, and his distal neurovascular exam is intact. Radiographs are normal. In order to prevent severe, subacute complications, further work-up is needed to rule out which of the following?

    A. peroneal nerve palsy

    B. popliteal artery injury

    C. medial collateral ligament disruption

    D. anterior cruciate ligament disruption

    E. dislocation of the patella

47. The lower leg of a 46-year-old factory worker is trapped when a piece of heavy machinery falls on it. Work-up in the emergency room reveals a swollen, painful leg, but radiographs are normal. She is admitted to the hospital for observation. Which of the following signs are indicative of an impending compartment syndrome?

    A. pain with passive motion of the toes

    B. intracompartmental pressures as high as 20 mm below diastolic blood pressure

   C. numbness and paresthesias of the foot
   D. increasing pain or pain seemingly out of proportion to the injury
   E. all of the above

48. A lateral tibial plateau fracture can occlude the anterior tibial artery and result in
   A. a pulseless but viable foot
   B. an undetectable vascular injury
   C. ischemic necrosis of the anterior tibial compartment
   D. paresthesias in the dorsum of the foot
   E. loss of plantar flexion reflex

49. In the hand, fractures of the phalanges usually do NOT require reduction unless
   A. an adjacent joint is dislocated
   B. the finger is particularly discolored and swollen
   C. an occult enchondroma is present in the bone
   D. the digit is badly deformed or unstable
   E. the patient is unable to wiggle the finger

DIRECTIONS (Questions 50 through 53): The group of questions below consists of lettered headings followed by a list of numbered words, phrases, or statements. For each numbered word, phrase, or statement, select the ONE lettered heading that is most closely associated with it. Each lettered heading may be used once, more than once, or not at all.

   A. sequestrum
   B. involucrum
   C. granulation tissue
   D. pseudoparalysis

50. Protective spasm immobilizing an involved extremity

51. Relative radiolucency of bone surrounding an osseous site of infection

52. Reactive osseous tissue deposited around a bone with osteomyelitis

53. Isolated necrotic bone within an abscess cavity

DIRECTIONS (Questions 54 through 58): Each of the questions or incomplete statements below is followed by five suggested answers or completions. Select the ONE that is best in each case.

---

54. A 13-year-old boy has a several day history of fever, malaise, and left distal thigh–knee pain. In addition to acute osteomyelitis, his differential diagnosis MUST include
    A. Ewing's sarcoma
    B. acute rheumatic fever
    C. leukemia
    D. acute septic arthritis
    E. all of the above

55. Which organism is MOST frequently encountered in hematogenous osteomyelitis?
    A. *Staphylococcus aureus*
    B. *Streptococcus*
    C. *Bacteroides*
    D. *Klebsiella*
    E. *Escherichia coli*

56. What organism is frequently associated with an osteomyelitis in patients with sickle cell disease?
    A. *S. aureus*
    B. *Streptococcus*
    C. *Salmonella*
    D. *Bacteroides*
    E. *E. coli*

57. After years of chronic infection, a sinus tract draining osteomyelitis may
    A. spontaneously and permanently heal
    B. develop squamous carcinoma
    C. change bacterial flora

    D. discharge granulomata
    E. become spontaneously painful

58. Aspiration of a joint with septic arthritis can reveal up to 200,000 white cells per cubic centimeter with what percentage of polymorphonuclear neutrophils?
    A. up to 50%
    B. up to 60%
    C. up to 70%
    D. up to 80%
    E. at least 90%

DIRECTIONS (Questions 59 through 62): The group of questions below consists of lettered headings followed by a list of numbered words, phrases, or statements. For each numbered word, phrase, or statement, select the ONE lettered heading that is most closely associated with it. Each lettered heading may be used once, more than once, or not at all.

    A. intralesional removal
    B. local resection
    C. wide local excision
    D. radical excision

59. Surgical removal of the entire anatomic compartment in which the tumor arises (frequently involves amputation)

60. Surgical removal of the tumor with a cuff of normal surrounding tissue

61. Surgical removal of the lesion intact through the capsule or reactive tissues surrounding it

62. Surgical removal involving curettage of the lesion from within

Orthopaedic Surgery

Answers and Comments

1. **(E)** In the treatment of fractures, the general rule is that the fragments, along with one proximal joint and one distal joint, should be immobilized. There are occasional exceptions to this rule, but in most instances both joints should be immobilized. (**Ref. 6,** pp. 1038, 1063)

2. **(C)** Numbness and paresthesias of the thumb and index finger are due to pressure on the median nerve. This nerve supplies those two digits. (**Ref. 6,** p. 1169)

3. **(C)** In treatment of both bone forearm fractures, the length, relationship, and curve of both bones must be exactly reproduced in order to restore wrist and forearm motion. In the adult, this ordinarily requires open reduction and plating of both fractures. In children with significant growth potential remaining, remodeling can correct significant angular (but not rotational) deformity or displacement. (**Ref. 6,** pp. 1036–1037)

4. **(D)** Extreme local tenderness over the suspected bone is a very helpful finding in the diagnosis of acute osteomyelitis in an infant. At this stage, within one week, x-rays of bone do not show any findings, and the adjoining joint may only show some effu-

sion. Blood cultures may be positive, but this may be part of septicemia. Constitutional disturbances are prominent, but may occur in septicemia alone. (**Ref. 6,** p. 1111)

5. **(E)** In a fall from a height, when a person lands on his feet, the fracture usually involves the calcaneus on one or both sides. If the force is severe, further injuries include central dislocation of the hip, fracture of the pelvis, and fracture of the spine. (**Ref. 6,** p. 1067)

6. **(C)** Typical deformity in a displaced fracture of the femoral neck is shortening and external rotation of the limb. Because of the fracture, the internal rotator muscles are no longer able to act, and the limb falls laterally by its weight and the unopposed action of the external rotators. (**Ref. 1,** pp. 1330–1331)

7. **(A)** Most dislocations of the hip are posterior dislocations, with the head riding on the dorsal surface of the ilium. The limb, in this situation, is usually flexed at the hip and abducted. (**Ref. 6,** p. 1047)

8. **(E)** Traditional treatment has usually required limb amputation, although more recent protocols include preoperative chemotherapy and sometimes reconstruction with allograft bone or, in the case of osteosarcomas about the knee, with fusion of the distal tibia to the proximal femur after rotating it 90 degrees so that the ankle can function as a knee (Van Ness rotationplasty). (**Ref. 6,** p. 1123)

9. **(B)** Of the carpal bones, the scaphoid is the one most frequently injured. Scaphoid fractures are often not visible on initial x-rays, and clinically suspicious wrists should be treated with wrist splints or casts for 1 to 2 weeks and the radiographs repeated. Untreated scaphoid fractures can have debilitating consequences. (**Ref. 6,** p. 1041)

10. **(C)** The most common serious complication after an open fracture is infection. Prevention requires surgical irrigation and debridement at the earliest opportunity, repeated every 58 to 72 hours until only clean, healthy tissue remains (usually a total of at least three surgeries). Broad spectrum prophylactic antibiotics are also required. (**Ref. 6,** p. 1115)

11. **(D)** Extensor plantar reflex is not a feature of lumbar disk protrusion. The protrusion affects the nerve root, and hence, it does not produce an upper motor neural lesion. The plantar reflex is usually absent. (**Ref. 6,** p. 1102)

12. **(B)** Mental deficiency is not a feature of achondroplasia; in fact, the individuals are fairly intelligent. (**Ref. 2,** p. 1892)

13. **(D)** Pyogenic arthritis is not common in young people active in sports. If these individuals have any injuries, they are usually traumatic synovitis or arthritis. (**Ref. 6,** p. 1119)

14. **(A)** The most frequent site of osteoarticular tuberculosis is the spine, and it is the lower thoracic and upper lumbar spine that is frequently affected. (**Ref. 6,** p. 1114)

15. **(B)** Spondylolysis is a bony defect in the neural arch. (**Ref. 2,** p. 1866)

16. **(D)** Spondylitis is a term for inflammatory disease of the spine. (**Ref. 2,** p. 1866)

17. **(C)** Spondylolisthesis is a slipping of one vertebra over the body of the next one located below. (**Ref. 2,** p. 1866)

18. **(A)** Spondylosis is the term used to describe the hypertrophic bone changes in which the spicules of bone project into the intervertebral foramen and may produce nerve root compression. (**Ref. 2,** p. 1865)

19. **(D)** Internal fixation of a fracture requires an open procedure that might increase the damage to the soft tissue. In addition, during internal fixation, there may be damage to the bone by the metallic plates and screws used. Because it is an open procedure, there is a risk of infection that can affect the bone and the material used for fixation. It is not essential in the treatment of all fractures. (**Ref. 2,** p. 1906)

20. **(D)** Indications for total hip replacement are osteoarthritis and rheumatoid arthritis. These produce gross limitation of movement and progress to fibrous ankylosis. Hip replacement is not advo-

cated in septic arthritis because of the risk of the prosthesis becoming infected. Gonococcal arthritis can usually be treated by medical measures. (**Ref. 6,** pp. 1050, 1119)

21. **(B)** Avascular necrosis of the femoral head develops in about 20% of patients with traumatic dislocation of the femoral head and is related to the amount of time spent in the dislocated position. Osteoarthritis occurs in about 50% of patients causing groin pain and decreased range of motion. (**Ref. 6,** p. 1047)

22. **(A)** Synovectomy in early rheumatoid arthritis is indicated for relief of pain. By removing the diseased synovial membranes, it slows down the inflammatory process that destroys tendons and joints and allows greater motion. Slowing down joint destruction also delays or eliminates the need for joint replacement. (**Ref. 6,** p. 1110)

23. **(E)** Diagnostic features of congenital dysplasia of the hip at birth include limitation of abduction of the hip when it is flexed, presence of Ortolani's sign (also called a "click"), and the apparent shortening of the thigh. Trendelenberg's sign cannot be seen until the child can stand on one leg. (**Ref. 6,** p. 1085)

24. **(C)** This child has congenital (dysplastic) spondylolisthesis. Other types include degenerative, traumatic, isthmic, and pathologic. Spondylolisthesis refers to the forward slip of a vertebra on the one below. The pars interarticularis, which is seen as the "neck of the scottie dog" is either elongated or fractured (spondylolysis) in the majority of these cases. (**Ref. 2,** pp. 1866–1867)

25. **(D)** Pathologic fractures of bones might occur in tumors, in developmental diseases of bone, and in a number of metabolic conditions. Congenital abnormalities that affect a single bone do not usually result in pathologic fracture. (**Ref. 2,** p. 1905)

26. **(D)** With this mechanism of injury, rupture of the anterior cruciate ligament of the knee is associated with medial collateral ligament damage. Meniscal tears, posterior cruciate ligament damage, or posterolateral corner disruption may also be associated, depending on the mechanism of injury. (**Ref. 6,** p. 1056)

27. **(B)** Immediate internal fixation gives the best chance for rapid recovery and avoidance of complications due to long enforced bedrest, necessary for the other treatments. (**Ref. 6,** p. 1052)

28. **(C)** Radial nerve injury produces wrist drop and inability to extend the hand. (**Ref. 6,** p. 1029)

29. **(D)** Isolated fractures of the fibula resulting from a direct blow are of little clinical consequence. They can usually be treated symptomatically with a brace or a cast for a week or two. When fibular shaft fractures are associated with ankle injuries, the management of these fractures frequently requires surgical intervention in order to restore the configuration of the talotibial joint. (**Ref. 6,** p. 1061)

30. **(C)** The sympathetic ganglia are located anterolateral to the vertebral bodies, and fractures of the thoracic and lumbar spine can result in a paralytic ileus. Bleeding from vertebral fractures into the retroperitoneal space may also produce a temporary ileus. (**Ref. 6,** p. 1014)

31. **(B)** Bones may fracture by repetitive bending movements. The fractures sustained from this accumulative minor trauma are called fatigue or stress fractures. They are frequently seen in military recruits and are called march fractures because they result from long training hikes. (**Ref. 6,** p. 1044)

32. **(A)** Fractures through the epiphyseal plate have been classified into a system of five grades of injury to help in the prognosis of possible future growth disturbance. All fractures of the epiphyses, no matter how minor, require a follow-up of a minimum of one year to monitor growth of the bone. (**Ref. 6,** p. 1073)

33. **(E)** Fat embolization following long bone fractures usually manifests itself within the first 12 to 72 hours. The typical clinical signs are a rising pulse and respiratory rate, tachypnea and dyspnea, petechiae, and confusion. The mental status changes are the result of a decreasing arterial PO_2. (**Ref. 6,** p. 195)

34. **(B)** A fracture through the pedicle of the axis (C2 vertebra) is known as a hangman's fracture. This traumatic spondylolisthesis

is the result of severe hyperextension of the neck, as produced in judicial hanging; a similar injury may be produced by an unrestrained motorist striking his or her chin on the steering wheel at the time of impact. (**Ref. 1,** p. 1296)

35. (**C**)   During the first 24 hours of spinal shock following a complete cord injury, total loss of motor and sensory function, including perianal sensation, is indicative of an ominous prognosis. Although the bulbocavernosus reflex may recover within the first 24 hours, it can return to function independently of the spinal cord from which it has been severed. (**Ref. 6,** p. 1013)

36. (**C**)   Anterior dislocation of the shoulder typically results from the arm's being in the posture of forced abduction, extension, and external rotation. In cases of chronic recurrent dislocations, an examiner may place the patient's extremity in this position, which will cause the patient to sense instability of his shoulder and impending dislocation. This is known as an "apprehension sign" because the patient is anxious that the shoulder will be inadvertently redislocated by this precarious posture of the arm. (**Ref. 6,** p. 1023)

37. (**D**)   Dislocation of the shoulder can injure the neural and vascular structures that pass by the glenohumeral joint. The axillary nerve is the most common neurovascular element injured by shoulder dislocation. Deltoid muscle function will be diminished, as well as sensation over the lateral aspect of the shoulder. Patients frequently recover from this nerve injury. (**Ref. 6,** p. 1024)

38. (**A**)   Fractures of the clavicle generally require only symptomatic treatment. Adults may be placed in a supportive figure-of-eight bandage, and infants frequently require no immobilization. In a polytrauma patient at bedrest, formal treatment is frequently unnecessary. Scapula fractures also can be managed by symptomatic relief. A simple arm sling to immobilize the shoulder blade may be helpful in the ambulatory patient. (**Ref. 6,** p. 1019)

39. (**A**)   The explanation is the same as for question 3. (**Ref. 6,** p. 1076)

40. (A) The brachial artery can be traumatized by a supracondylar fracture of the humerus. This requires emergent reduction and stabilization of the fracture, with restoration of blood flow. If untreated, profound ischemia of the forearm will ensue with subsequent contracture of the hand. (**Ref. 6,** p. 1075)

41. (E) In toddlers, subluxation of the radial head through the annular ligament at the elbow can be produced by a friend or parent impatiently tugging on the child's arm. This painful condition is known as a "pulled elbow," or more commonly, "nursemaid's elbow." Frequently, the temporary subluxation is reduced when the x-ray technician places the child's arm on the x-ray film for a radiograph. Symptomatic treatment in a sling usually results in a prompt recovery of full function in a few days. (**Ref. 6,** p. 1076)

42. (D) These are the three components of a clubfoot deformity, each of which may vary in severity. There are many other pediatric foot deformities. Some, like flatfoot or intoeing, rarely require treatment. (**Ref. 6,** p. 1090)

43. (E) A blood clot beneath the fingernail is exquisitely painful, and this subungual hematoma can be decompressed by trephining the fingernail. A hole can be made in the nail plate by painting it with antiseptic solution and searing a hole through it with a heated paper clip. Relief of symptoms is prompt. (**Ref. 4,** p.118)

44. (A) Massive hemorrhage is a common complication of fractures of the pelvis, resulting in hypotension. It can be confused with an acute abdomen. Sometimes the bladder, rectum, and sciatic nerve are injured by pelvic fractures, but this is less common than massive blood loss. The treatment described reduces pelvic volume and helps to control blood loss into this region. (**Ref. 4,** p. 149; **Ref. 6,** p. 1018)

45. (B) The patient who has sustained a fracture of the femur may lose 2 to 3 units of blood within the fracture site. If the patient has sustained bilateral fractured femurs, then blood loss can be 4 to 6 units of blood. Patients with bilateral fractures of the femur and pelvic fractures may require large amounts of blood replacement because of hemorrhage within the fracture sites. (**Ref. 1,** p. 1333)

46. (B) Almost half of patients who sustain a dislocation of the knee will have a popliteal artery injury. This vascular injury is usually the result of hyperextension of the knee at the time of injury. Vascular evaluation and monitoring of the blood flow of a limb that has sustained a dislocation of the knee is imperative. (**Ref. 6,** p. 1056)

47. (E) Compartment tissue pressures can be measured by several different methods. In general, tissue perfusion decreases significantly when the compartment pressure approaches a level of 20 mm below diastolic pressure. At this time, fasciotomy is required to restore microcirculation of blood. (**Ref. 6,** p. 1063)

48. (C) The anterior tibial artery supplies the structures of the anterior compartment of the leg. The anterior tibial pulse is usually absent although back flow from collateral circulation may create a palpable pulse distal to the block. Ischemia of the anterior compartment of the leg causes weakness of foot inversion and ankle dorsiflexion, and may cause numbness and paresthesias of the first dorsal web space. (**Ref. 1,** p. 1336; **Ref. 4,** p. 149)

49. (D) Fractures of the phalanges usually do not require reduction unless badly deformed or grossly unstable. Most fractures of the phalanges can be treated by simple buddy taping to the adjacent digit to restore the natural alignment of the finger. The goal of treatment is to restore motion and the side-by-side posture of the digits for the proper finger stance during grasp. (**Ref. 6,** p. 1173)

50. (D) Protective muscle spasm in the involved extremity of a patient, particularly children, with septic arthritis will produce an involuntary "pseudoparalysis." This can be a very dramatic physical finding in an agitated and combative child who is flailing three extremities while leaving the involved extremity motionless on the examining table. (**Ref. 1,** pp. 1354–1355)

51. (C) In a bone infection, the zone of relative radiolucency surrounding the site of osteomyelitis is produced by the ingrowth of granulation tissue. This early attempt at healing is only evident upon x-ray about 12 to 14 days following the onset of the focus of infection. (**Ref. 1,** p. 1351)

52. **(B)**   Reactive osseous tissue that is deposited around a site of osteomyelitis is called involucrum. This is the response of a host bone to wall off and repair the focus of infection. (**Ref. 1,** p. 1351)

53. **(A)**   In osteomyelitis, a focus of pus under pressure can cause ischemic necrosis of bone. The necrotic bone within the abscess cavity is called a sequestrum. This dead piece of bone will serve as a foreign body and facilitate the infection. Debridement of the sequestrum is part of the routine care of osteomyelitis. (**Ref. 1,** p. 1351)

54. **(E)**   Ewing's sarcoma, acute rheumatic fever, leukemia, and septic arthritiscan all mimic acute osteomyelitis. Lab tests, radiographs, bone and indium scans, and MRI may all be helpful in making the diagnosis. (**Ref. 1,** p. 1352; **Ref. 6,** p. 1111)

55. **(A)**   Although all of the organisms listed may cause osteomyelitis, *Staphylococcus aureus* is the most common. In neonates, Group B streptococcus is also common, and in toddlers *Haemophilus influenzae* is a frequent offender. (**Ref. 6,** p. 1111)

56. **(C)**   When patients with sickle cell anemia contract osteomyelitis, infection of the bone with *Salmonella* may be seen. The exact cause of this unusual infectious agent is not clearly understood, but it must be borne in mind when treating these patients. (**Ref. 6,** p. 1111)

57. **(B)**   In patients with chronic osteomyelitis that has been draining for decades, the sinus tract is lined with squamous epithelium. In longstanding cases, this squamous epithelium may undergo metaplasia into a squamous carcinoma. This is sometimes signaled by an unusual change in the nature of the chronic drainage. A radical surgery, including amputation, is sometimes required. (**Ref. 6,** p. 1117)

58. **(E)**   Aspiration of a septic joint will produce pus with a cell count of 50,000 to 200,000 white cells per cubic centimeter. One of the hallmarks of the differential white cell count is the presence of at least 90% polymorphonuclear leukocytes. Inflammatory synovitis, as seen in rheumatoid arthritis and the crystalline

arthropathies, can sometime produce alarmingly high cell counts; but the differential count of polymorphonuclear leukocytes is much lower, indicating a chronic process. (**Ref. 6,** p. 1119)

59. (**D**)   Radical excision of a musculoskeletal tumor requires removal of the entire anatomic compartment in which the lesion arises. This ablative surgery frequently requires amputation of the limb. (**Ref. 1,** p. 1359)

60. (**C**)   Wide local excision of a musculoskeletal tumor requires removal of the lesion with a cuff of several centimeters of normal surrounding tissue. This type of surgical extirpation is usually part of a limb-salvaging procedure. (**Ref. 1,** p. 1359)

61. (**B**)   Local resection of a musculoskeletal tumor requires removal of the mass intact through the pseudocapsule or reactive tissue surrounding the lesion. This type of resection is suited to benign lesions that have less chance of recurrence. (**Ref. 1,** p. 1359)

62. (**A**)   Intralesional removal of a musculoskeletal tumor involves curettage of the lesion from within. In general, benign lesions sometimes require no treatment if they are asymptomatic, but they may require intralesional removal if they are painful. (**Ref. 6,** p. 1121)

11

Cardiothoracic Surgery
Richard A. Schmaltz

DIRECTIONS (Questions 1 through 43): Each of the questions or incomplete statements below is followed by five suggested answers or completions. Select the ONE that is best in each case.

---

1. The MOST common nonbacterial organism causing endocarditis is
   - **A.** cryptococcosis
   - **B.** aspergillosis
   - **C.** actinomycosis
   - **D.** candidiasis
   - **E.** histoplasmosis

2. All the following indicate situations that are associated with spontaneous pneumothorax EXCEPT
   - **A.** young adult males who smoke cigarettes
   - **B.** initial treatment usually by tube thoracostomy (chest tube)
   - **C.** pleural gas reabsorption facilitated by oxygen supplementation
   - **D.** rapid reexpansion of a complete pneumothorax occasionally causing ipsilateral pulmonary edema
   - **E.** rarely recurring after the first event (less than 10%)

3. Mesotheliomas of the pleura are characterized by all of the following EXCEPT
  A. they are the most common primary tumors of the pleura
  B. they may be localized or diffuse
  C. they may be benign or malignant
  D. histologically, they may be fibrous or epithelioid
  E. they can be easily classified pathologically and differentiated from other carcinomas

4. The most common site of metastasis from carcinoma of the lung is
  A. bone
  B. adrenal gland
  C. liver
  D. kidney
  E. hilar and mediastinal lymph nodes

5. The most common symptom of bronchogenic carcinoma is
  A. bone pain
  B. hemoptysis
  C. chest pain
  D. dyspnea
  E. cough

6. Evidence of incurability at the time of surgical exploration for bronchogenic carcinoma include all of the following EXCEPT
  A. cardiac metastasis
  B. pleural fluid positive for tumor cells
  C. extension of tumor onto the aorta
  D. invasion of the tumor into the pericardium
  E. localized chest wall involvement

7. The one-year survival for untreated bronchogenic carcinoma is
  A. 40%
  B. 30%
  C. 20%
  D. 15%
  E. 5%

8. The MOST common tumor of the chest wall is
    A. chondrosarcoma
    B. plasmacytoma
    C. osteogenic sarcoma
    D. Ewing's sarcoma
    E. metastatic tumor

9. The agent most commonly identified with mediastinal fibrosis is
    A. tuberculosis
    B. collagen vascular disease
    C. histoplasmosis
    D. chronic bacterial infection
    E. blastomycosis

10. The most common cause of mediastinal hemorrhage
    A. bleeding from tumor
    B. "spontaneous" following severe coughing
    C. dissecting thoracic aneurysm
    D. anticoagulation therapy
    E. trauma

11. The most common cause of superior vena cava syndrome is
    A. lymphoma
    B. thymoma
    C. thyroid tumor
    D. idiopathic mediastinal fibrosis
    E. bronchogenic carcinoma

12. All of the following statements are true of thymomas EXCEPT
    A. they represent one of the most common mediastinal tumors
    B. they are associated with myasthenia gravis
    C. they usually appear in adult life
    D. they may appear as small circumscribed lesions or as ill-defined lobulated masses
    E. they are always benign

13. The MOST common pericardial tumor is
    A. teratoma
    B. lymphoma

C. mesothelioma
D. metastatic bronchogenic carcinoma
E. hemangiomas

14. Catheterization of the right heart will show a characteristic "square root" or a "dip-and-plateau" configuration of the diastolic pressure with
A. congestive heart failure
B. cardiomyopathy
C. cardiac tamponade
D. constrictive pericarditis
E. myocardial ischemia

15. In regard to intracardiac shunts, mixing of the saturated arterial and desaturated venous blood on the right side of the circulation and increase in pulmonary blood flow relative to systemic flow (left-to-right shunt) is associated with the following EXCEPT
A. ventricular septal defects (VSD)
B. patent ductus arteriosus (PDA)
C. atrial septal defect (ASD)
D. aortopulmonary window
E. tetralogy of Fallot

16. Longstanding severe left-to-right shunting can lead to irreversible pulmonary hypertension, causing a right-to-left shunt. This disease state is known as
A. Kussmaul's sign
B. Eisenmenger's syndrome
C. Starling relation
D. Wolff–Parkinson–White syndrome
E. Prinzmetal's syndrome

17. Occlusion of which of the major coronary arteries poses the MOST serious risk for morbidity and mortality?
A. left anterior descending artery
B. obtuse marginal artery
C. left main coronary artery
D. right coronary artery
E. circumflex artery

18. Percutaneous transluminal coronary angioplasty reduces athero-sclerotic stenosis by producing a "controlled injury" of the arterial wall with intimal fracture and medial splitting and stretching. Recurrent stenosis (loss of 50% or more of the initial diameter gain) occurs in what percentage of patients?
    A. 10%
    B. 20%
    C. 30%
    D. 40%
    E. 50%

19. The MOST effective drug used in the treatment of cardiac arrest is
    A. sodium bicarbonate
    B. calcium chloride
    C. atropine sulfate
    D. dopamine
    E. epinephrine

20. The usual dose of lidocaine used to control life-threatening dys-rhythmia is
    A. 50- to 100-mg bolus and 1 to 3 mg/min drip
    B. 200- to 300-mg bolus and 5 mg/min drip
    C. 400- to 500-mg bolus and 5 to 8 mg/min drip
    D. 600- to 800-mg bolus and 5 to 8 mg/min drip
    E. 1000-mg bolus and 8 to 10 mg/min drip

21. The ductus arteriosus connects which anatomical structures?
    A. right pulmonary artery to the aortic arch
    B. main pulmonary trunk to the innominate artery
    C. left pulmonary artery to the arch just beyond the subclavian take-off
    D. left pulmonary artery to the left subclavian artery
    E. main pulmonary artery to the right subclavian artery

22. All of the following are true of coarctation of the aorta EXCEPT
    A. it is classified as preductal or postductal
    B. the aortic valve is frequently bicuspid
    C. it is associated with an essentially normal life span

D. most cases can be diagnosed by the difference in arterial pulsations and blood pressure, comparing the upper to lower extremities

E. the classic chest x-ray has a "3" sign

23. All of the following statements are true regarding ventricular septal defects EXCEPT

A. many (25% to 50%) will close spontaneously during childhood

B. the hemodynamic state in patients with a large ventricular septal defect (VSD) depends upon the pulmonary vascular resistance

C. pulmonary vascular resistance greater than 12 Wood units is considered inoperable

D. a systolic thrill is felt over the precordium

E. infants are usually most symptomatic during the first few days of life

24. All of the following are characteristics of tetralogy of Fallot EXCEPT

A. cyanosis

B. boot-shaped heart (coeur en sabot) on chest x-ray

C. unexplained bleeding tendency

D. clubbing of the fingers and toes (hypertrophic pulmonary osteoarthropathy)

E. anemia (mild)

25. The LEAST helpful procedure to improve or correct the symptoms of transposition of the great arteries is

A. balloon atrial septostomy (Rashkind)

B. palliative atrial septectomy (Blalock)

C. repositioning of the great arteries over their appropriate ventricles

D. diversion of venous inflow at the atrial level (Mustard), ie, creation of an intra-atrial baffle to redirect systemic and pulmonary venous return

E. creation of two large interatrial channels for crossing the systemic and pulmonary circulations (Senning)

26. Indications for surgical resection of a left ventricular aneurysm include all of the following EXCEPT
 A. congestive heart failure
 B. angina
 C. intractable dysrhythmia
 D. risk of spontaneous rupture
 E. systemic emboli

27. Complications of severe mitral stenosis include all of the following EXCEPT
 A. low cardiac output causing fatigue
 B. atrial dysrhythmia
 C. left ventricular enlargement
 D. systemic embolization
 E. pulmonary vascular engorgement and hypertension causing dyspnea

28. The MOST common primary cardiac tumor is
 A. rhabdomyosarcoma
 B. angiosarcoma
 C. fibrosarcoma
 D. myxoma
 E. leiomyosarcoma

29. The MOST common site for myxoma to be found is the
 A. left atrium
 B. right atrium
 C. left ventricle
 D. right ventricle
 E. interventricular septum

30. Indications for permanent pacing include all of the following EXCEPT
 A. sick sinus syndrome and bradytachyarrhythmia
 B. complete atrioventricular (AV) block
 C. Mobitz type I AV block
 D. symptomatic bifascicular and trifascicular block
 E. intractable low cardiac output syndrome benefitted by temporary pacing

31. A 60-year-old male patient presents with exertional angina and has recently had an episode of syncope after moderate exercise. On physical exam he was found to have delayed carotid upstroke and a grade III–IV/VI systolic murmur heard best over the second right intercostal space with radiation to the neck. Chest x-ray shows mild cardiomegaly, and electrocardiogram (ECG) shows left ventricular hypertrophy and an old inferior myocardial infarction. Cardiac catheterization shows a 60-mm pressure gradient across the aortic valve with a valve area of one square cm. Coronary catheterization revealed 100% occlusion of a small right coronary system, an unremarkable circumflex, and a 70% occlusion proximal left interior descending artery. The next step would be

A. digitalization and diuretic therapy with follow-up in 6 months
B. captopril (after load-reducing agent) and diuretic therapy with follow-up in 6 months
C. percutaneous balloon valvuloplasty
D. aortic valve replacement only
E. aortic valve replacement and coronary artery bypass

32. A 55-year-old male presents with exertional dyspnea and orthopnea (New York Heart Association, class III). Physical examination reveals a grade III–IV/VI holosystolic murmur at the cardiac apex radiating into the axilla. The chest x-ray shows moderate cardiomegaly. The ventricular ejection fraction is 50% by radionuclide ventriculography. The patient has atrial fibrillation with a controlled ventricular response. Which of the following is the MOST appropriate management in this situation?

A. captopril (after load-reducing agent) and diuretic therapy with follow-up in 6 months
B. digitalization and long term anticoagulation with yearly follow-up
C. 2 weeks of anticoagulation followed by electrical cardioversion
D. mitral valve replacement or repair
E. coronary arteriography to assess the status of coronary arteries, followed by mitral valve repair or replacement

33. The most common cause of lung abscess is
  A. aspiration of septic material from the mouth or oropharynx
  B. blood-borne infection
  C. lymphatic spread
  D. penetrating injury of the chest
  E. bronchogenic carcinoma

34. The most common site of lung abscess is the
  A. left upper lobe
  B. left lower lobe
  C. lingular segment
  D. superior and posterior segments of the right lung
  E. right middle lobe

35. The BEST treatment of hemothorax with 500 cc or more of blood in the pleural space is
  A. needle aspiration
  B. closed thoracostomy and tube drainage
  C. thoracotomy and ligation of bleeding vessel(s)
  D. wait and watch
  E. transfusion of fresh blood

36. The MOST common cause of empyema is
  A. pneumonic process in the underlying lung
  B. rupture of an emphysematous bulla
  C. penetrating injury of the chest
  D. subphrenic abscess
  E. rupture of the thoracic esophagus

37. All of the following are indications for resection treatment in pulmonary tuberculosis EXCEPT
  A. an open cavity with positive sputum after 3 to 6 months of chemotherapy
  B. patients with negative sputum with residual destroyed segment
  C. localized infection with atypical acid-fast organisms
  D. fresh lesion with positive sputum
  E. tuberculous bronchiectasis of middle and lower lobes

38. A helpful finding on the chest x-ray to make a diagnosis of chronic constrictive pericarditis is
A. small heart
B. displacement of the right bronchus
C. prominent hilar markings of the lungs
D. calcification of the pericardium
E. elevated dome of the diaphragm

39. The MAJOR contraindication for surgical treatment of a patent ductus arteriosus is
A. left-to-right shunt
B. shunt from aorta to pulmonary artery
C. shunt from pulmonary artery to aorta
D. cardiomegaly
E. hilar dance on fluoroscopy of chest

40. All of the following features are diagnostic of tetralogy of Fallot EXCEPT
A. stunted growth
B. long, narrow fingers
C. thrill in the precordial region
D. harsh systolic murmur along left sternal border
E. cyanosis of fingertips

41. Aneurysms of the ascending aorta may be due to all of the following EXCEPT
A. Marfan's syndrome
B. trauma
C. syphilis
D. atherosclerosis
E. Erdheim's cystic medial necrosis

42. The most frequent and significant effect of an aneurysm of the ascending aorta is
A. rupture
B. aortic valvular insufficiency
C. erosion of sternum
D. pressure on the trachea
E. pressure on the vena cava

43. An etiologic factor in the development of pleural mesothelioma is
   A. pneumoconiosis
   B. asbestosis
   C. anthracosis
   D. genetic predisposition
   E. collagen vascular disease

DIRECTIONS (Questions 44 through 55): Each group of questions below consists of lettered headings followed by a list of numbered words, phrases, or statements. For each numbered word, phrase, or statement, select the ONE lettered heading that is most closely associated with it. Each lettered heading may be used once, more than once, or not at all.

Questions 44 through 47

Match the findings on auscultation with the abnormality.

   A. ventricular septal defect (VSD)
   B. atrial septal defect (ASD)
   C. patent ductus arteriosus (PDA)
   D. tetralogy of Fallot

44. Split-second heart sound in all phases of respiration

45. Continuous, rumbling murmur

46. Loud systolic murmur along the left sternal border

47. Loud systolic murmur along the left sternal border and over the pulmonary artery

Questions 48 through 51

   A. histoplasmosis
   B. coccidioidomycosis
   C. North American blastomycosis
   D. aspergillosis

48. Occurrence of thin-walled cavities and suppuration in lung

49. Cutaneous lesion

50. Fungus ball in the lung

51. Solitary nodule in the lung

Questions 52 through 55

    A. anterior mediastinum
    B. superior mediastinum
    C. posterior mediastinum
    D. middle mediastinum

52. Thymoma

53. Teratoma

54. Pericardial cyst

55. Neurogenic tumor

DIRECTIONS (Questions 56 and 57): This section consists of a clinical situation followed by a series of questions. Study the situation and select the ONE best answer to each question following it.

A 60-year-old, 100-kg man with a 60 pack-year smoking history is evaluated for cough and occasional minimal hemoptysis. His review of systems is otherwise unremarkable. A chest x-ray reveals a 2-cm nodule in the midportion of the right upper lobe. A comparison film from four years ago shows no abnormality.

56. What is the probability that this lesion represents a carcinoma?
    A. 15%
    B. 35%
    C. 55%
    D. 75%
    E. 90%

57. Which of the following studies preclude surgical resection?
- **A.** CT scan of the abdomen showing a 2-cm right adrenal mass
- **B.** FEV_1 of 1.5 liters
- **C.** $Paco_2$ of 50 torr
- **D.** Pao_2 of 70 torr on room air
- **E.** CT scan of the chest showing a 1.5-cm right paratracheal lymph node

---

DIRECTIONS (Questions 58 through 60): Each of the questions or incomplete statements below is followed by five suggested answers or completions. Select the ONE that is best in each case.

---

58. A 20-year-old male was injured in a head-on motor vehicle collision. He is found to have a flail right chest. His blood pressure is 130/90; pulse 98. The chest x-ray shows early pulmonary contusion but no effusion or pneumothorax. He was initially cooperative but is becoming increasingly agitated and dyspneic and complains of severe pain when breathing. His respiratory rate is 40 and his Pao_2 is 70 torr on a 70% face mask. Appropriate therapy would be
- **A.** 20 mg morphine IM to control pain so he could breath more easily
- **B.** increasing the Fio_2 to 100% and repeating blood gas in one hour
- **C.** infusing one to three L of Ringer's lactate to increase his circulatory volume.
- **D.** intubation and mechanical ventilation
- **E.** taking the patient to the operating room to mechanically stabilize the fracture segment

59. The MOST common congenital deformity of the chest wall is
- **A.** pectus excavatum
- **B.** sternal fissure
- **C.** Poland's syndrome
- **D.** pectus carinatum
- **E.** absence of the lower ribs associated with a hemivertebra

60. A 65-year-old diabetic male, who has been a heavy smoker and is moderately obese, undergoes an emergent aortocoronary bypass procedure performed for unstable angina. Both the right and left internal mammary arteries were utilized because of lack of adequate vein conduit. Initially, the cardiac indices were poor (cardiac index 2.2), and he required moderate inotropic support. He improved and by the third postoperative day was extubated and all inotropic support was able to be discontinued. He was discharged on the seventh postoperative day. He now presents 12 days postoperatively with constant, diffuse, central chest pain, and spiking fever to 102°F. Examination of the incisions shows no sign of infection. His lungs are clear to examination. He has no dysuria or abdominal pain. His laboratory data reveals a white count of 18,000 with a left shift. The MOST concerning probable diagnosis is

A. urinary tract infection
B. cytomegalovirus infection from blood transfusion
C. mediastinitis
D. urinary tract infection
E. intra-abdominal abscess

Cardiothoracic Surgery

Answers and Comments

1. **(D)** The most common infecting organism causing nonbacterial endocarditis is *Candida*. Some cases of *Aspergillus* have also been reported. Several contributory factors have been identified—prolonged antibiotic therapy, indwelling catheters, and compromised immune state found in patients who have undergone bypass. (**Ref. 1**, p. 1715)

2. **(E)** The incidence of recurrence of a spontaneous pneumothorax in the young adult (20 to 40 years old) is 50%; the incidence after the second event is 60%, and after the third event is 80% or more. Therefore, most surgeons advocate a definitive surgical procedure (oversewing of the blebs and pleural abrasion) after the second event. (**Ref. 1**, p. 1721; **Ref. 3**, p. 686)

3. **(E)** Malignant mesothelioma is a locally aggressive tumor that has a very poor prognosis. Histologically, mesothelioma can present as either fibrous or fibrosarcomatous and an epithelioid variety. Mixtures of these histologic types in both benign and malignant lesions make differentiation of this tumor difficult. (**Ref. 1**, p. 2073; **Ref. 2**, p. 991; **Ref. 3**, p. 683)

4. **(E)** The most common site of metastasis of primary carcinoma of the lung is to the lymph nodes in the hilum and the mediastinum. Spread to other organs (in order of incidence): bones, adrenal glands, liver, kidneys, heart, and contralateral lung. (**Ref. 1**, p. 1748; **Ref. 2**, p. 1007; **Ref. 3**, p. 729)

5. **(E)** The most common symptom of bronchogenic carcinoma is cough. It occurs in 75% of patients. Hemoptysis is seen in about 30% of patients. Severe chest pain usually signifies chest wall invasion. Dyspnea is associated with obstruction of major bronchi. (**Ref. 1,** p. 1749; **Ref. 2,** p. 1000; **Ref. 3,** pp. 727–728)

6. **(E)** At the time of exploratory thoracotomy, spread of tumor involving the parietal pleura, pericardium, heart, or other mediastinal structures is generally a sign of incurability. Long-term survivors have been reported with en bloc resection of the tumor and chest wall. (**Ref. 1,** p. 1753; **Ref. 2,** p. 1003)

7. **(E)** The one-year survival rate for *untreated* carcinoma of the lung is only 5%. (**Ref. 2,** p. 1006)

8. **(E)** The most common tumor of the chest wall is metastatic, usually from the lung or breast. Benign primary tumors include chondromas, osteochondromas, bone cysts, fibrous dysplasia, and eosinophilic granulomas. Malignant primary tumors are chondrosarcoma, fibrosarcoma, osteogenic sarcoma, Ewing's carcinoma, and myeloma. (**Ref. 1,** p. 1764; **Ref. 3,** pp. 669–670)

9. **(C)** Histoplasmosis is identified as an agent causing fibrosing mediastinitis. (**Ref. 2,** p. 985; **Ref. 3,** p. 763)

10. **(E)** The most common cause of mediastinal hemorrhage is trauma. Other causes are thoracic aortic dissection, rupture of aortic aneurysms, or surgical procedures within the thorax. (**Ref. 1,** p. 1774; **Ref. 2,** p. 1023)

11. **(E)** Most superior vena cava syndromes are secondary to invasive malignancy. Bronchogenic carcinoma, frequently from the right upper lobe, is the most common tumor. Thymic and thyroid tumors are less frequently responsible. Less than 25% of patients will have a benign process such as fibrosing mediastinitis, thoracic aortic aneurysm, or caval thrombosis due to an indwelling catheter or instrumentation. (**Ref. 1,** p. 1774; **Ref. 2,** p. 1023; **Ref. 3,** p. 763)

12. **(E)** A significant number of thymomas are malignant (>30%). The establishment of malignancy is difficult histologically and is more readily documented by direct invasion of mediastinal tissues as noted during operation. The staging of malignant thymomas is as follows: Stage I—encapsulated, stage 2—pericapsular growth, stage III—invasive of adjacent organs, and stage IV—extrathoracic spread. The five-year survival in these patients is stage dependent: Stage I—85% to 100%, stage II—60% to 80%, stage III—40% to 70%, and stage IV—50%. (**Ref. 1,** p. 1786; **Ref. 2,** pp. 1038–1039; **Ref. 3,** pp. 753–755)

13. **(D)** The most common tumor of the pericardium is metastatic, most frequently bronchogenic. Breast cancer, as well as leukemia and lymphoma, also commonly metastasize to the pericardium. Of the primary neoplasms of the pericardium, mesothelioma is the most frequent malignant neoplasm. Approximately half of pericardial neoplasms are benign, including teratomas, hemangiomas, leiomyofibromas, lipomas, and fibromas. (**Ref. 1,** p. 1823; **Ref. 2,** p. 1051; **Ref. 3,** p. 755)

14. **(D)** During right-sided cardiac catheterization in patients with pericardial constriction, a "square root" or "dip-and-plateau" configuration of the diastolic pressure wave is characteristic. This configuration is not seen in patients with cardiac tamponade, although both typically produce elevation and equalization of the right and left ventricular diastolic pressure. Because of continuous compression of the heart in patients with tamponade, one typically sees a slow, early diastolic filling and an attenuated atrial Y descent. Pulsus paradoxus is seen with tamponade because negative intrathoracic pressure during inspiration enhances right heart filling at the expense of left heart filling. (**Ref. 1,** p. 1830; **Ref. 3,** p. 895)

15. **(E)** The disorders of VSD, PDA, ASD, and aortopulmonary window all classically produce left-to-right shunts. The uncomplicated tetralogy of Fallot is a right-to-left shunt, with desaturated blood entering the systemic circulation, causing cyanosis. These patients often have severe anoxia (arterial oxygen saturation of 35% to 85%), causing compensatory polycythemia and eventual clubbing of the extremities. (**Ref. 1,** p. 1910; **Ref. 3,** p. 812)

16. **(B)**   Severe left-to-right shunting causes pulmonary hypertension. In some unfortunate patients, pulmonary hypertension can lead to irreversible pulmonary and vascular changes with increased resistance. At that point, the shunt reverses with a right-to-left shunt, which produces an inoperable situation know as Eisenmenger's syndrome. Kussmaul's sign is the increase in venous pressure during inspiration, which is reflected by visual evidence of increased jugular venous distention in patients with constrictive pericarditis. The Starling relation states that if the filling (preload) of the heart is increased, the heart will contract more forcefully. Wolff–Parkinson–White syndrome is an example of a reentrant arrhythmia where there is one or more anomalous atrial–ventricular connections that cause a short PR interval and a wide QRS complex due to eccentric and premature activation of the ventricles during sinus rhythm. A life-threatening tachycardia can ensue. Prinzmetal's syndrome, also known as variant angina, is felt to be due to coronary artery spasm. People with this syndrome are noted to have ST segment elevation during periods of ischemia. (**Ref. 1,** p. 1901; **Ref. 3,** p. 803)

17. **(C)**   In most individuals, the left side of the coronary anatomy originates from one major vessel called the left main coronary. From this short vessel, the left anterior descending and the circumflex systems originate. A significant lesion of this short trunk causes the patient to be at high risk for major infarction and death. (**Ref. 1,** p. 1959; **Ref. 2,** pp. 1117–1118)

18. **(C)**   Most series indicate that there is a 30% recurrence of significant stenosis following percutaneous transluminal coronary artery angioplasty. (**Ref. 1,** p. 1841; **Ref. 3,** p. 887)

19. **(E)**   All of the drugs mentioned are important adjuvants in patients who require cardiac resuscitation. However, epinephrine is by far the most effective; its primary benefit appears to be its vasoconstrictive effect. (**Ref. 2,** p. 1182; **Ref. 3,** p. 854)

20. **(A)**   Lidocaine is the most common drug used for acute antiarrhythmic control for acute dysrhythmia. The usual dose is a 50- to 100-mg bolus, followed by a 1- to 3-mg/min drip. The loading dose can be repeated in 10 minutes if the dysrhythmia persists. Second-line drugs include a bretylium 300-mg bolus or a slow infusion of procainamide. (**Ref. 1,** p. 1848; **Ref. 3,** p. 850)

21. **(C)**   Patent ductus arteriosus is one of the most common congenital heart defects. A ductus arteriosus connects the left pulmonary artery to the aortic arch just beyond the subclavian take-off. In utero, blood ejected by the ventricles flows almost exclusively through the ductus to the lower extremities and placenta, bypassing the lungs. At birth, expansion of the lungs decreases the pulmonary vascular resistance, allowing blood to flow from the main pulmonary artery through the smaller vessels of the lung circulation. (**Ref. 1,** p. 1855; **Ref. 2,** p. 1061; **Ref. 3,** pp. 807–808)

22. **(C)**   Coarctation of the aorta is a significant localized narrowing of the aorta. It occurs in 10% to 15% of congenital heart disease cases. It is more common in males (3:1). Death occurs from rupture of the aorta, cardiac failure, rupture of intracranial aneurysms and bacterial endocarditis. If untreated, the life expectancy is generally reduced by half. (**Ref. 1,** pp. 1859–1860; **Ref. 2,** pp. 1065–1067; **Ref. 3,** pp. 787–789)

23. **(E)**   In early infancy, most neonates have a moderately elevated pulmonary vascular resistance because of persistence of the medial thickening of the small pulmonary arteries normally present in the fetus. During the first few weeks of life, the pulmonary vessels mature, which results in the decrease of pulmonary resistance. Therefore, the magnitude of the left-to-right shunt increases tremendously, at which time symptoms develop. (**Ref. 1,** pp. 1901–1902; **Ref. 2,** pp. 1085–1086)

24. **(E)**   Patients with tetralogy of Fallot usually have a high hematocrit (as great as 90%) due to severe anoxia and resultant erythrocytosis. (**Ref. 1,** p. 1911; **Ref. 2,** p. 1090, **Ref. 3**, p. 814)

25. **(B)**   Transposition of the great vessels is incompatible with life unless there is a concomitant intracirculatory shunt (ASD, VSD, PDA, bronchial vessel-to-pulmonary shunt). A decision as to the type of repair must be made early on. This generally involves either a repositioning of the transposed arteries (arterial switch) or diversion of the venous inflow at the atrial level (Mustard or Senning). A balloon septostomy, as described by Rashkind, can increase mixing of venous and oxygenated blood at the atrial level in order to palliate an infant until he or she matures to the point when a definitive procedure can be done. (**Ref. 1,** p. 1943; **Ref. 3,** p. 821)

26. **(D)** The usual indications for a resection of a left ventricular aneurysm include congestive heart failure, angina, dysrhythmia, and peripheral emboli (which occur rarely). Rupture does not usually occur with this type of aneurysm. (**Ref. 1,** pp. 1986–1987; **Ref. 2,** p. 1125; **Ref. 3,** pp. 892–893)

27. **(C)** The left ventricle is usually small in patients with severe mitral stenosis because there is decreased blood flow due to valve restriction. Patients with fixed mitral stenosis cannot increase their cardiac output with exercise—this is one of the etiologies of the associated fatigue. Atrial dysrhythmia (fibrillation) is frequently seen and is probably due to atrial dilation and alteration in normal atrial conduction pathways. Pulmonary venous hypertension is caused by valve obstruction. The result is distention and thickening of the pulmonary capillaries; intimal fibrosis of the pulmonary veins and arterioles can also be seen. Systemic embolization is present in 25% of patients. (**Ref. 1,** p. 2029; **Ref. 2,** p. 1144; **Ref. 3,** p. 857)

28. **(D)** Primary cardiac tumors are rare, and the majority are benign. The most common type is a benign myxoma. (**Ref. 1,** p. 2071; **Ref. 2,** p. 1163; **Ref. 3,** p. 882)

29. **(A)** Seventy-five percent of myxomas originate in the left atrium, and 20% occur in the right atrium. The majority of these arise from the region of the fossa ovalis. (**Ref. 1,** p. 2071; **Ref. 2,** p. 1164; **Ref. 3,** p. 882)

30. **(C)** Mobitz type I AV block is not an indication for permanent pacing. The indications are: sick sinus syndrome, bradytachyarrhythmia syndrome, Mobitz type II AV block that is symptomatic, complete A-V block, symptomatic bilateral bundle branch block, bifascicular or incomplete trifascicular block with intermittent complete AV block following acute myocardial infarction, carotid sinus syncope, recurrent drug-resistant tachyarrhythmia improved by temporary pacing, and intractable low cardiac output syndrome benefitted by temporary pacing. (**Ref. 1,** p. 2077; **Ref. 2,** p. 1170)

31. **(E)** The patient has significant aortic valve stenosis as measured by the gradient across the valve, as well as the reduced valve area.

The main indications for operation are the development of angina, congestive heart failure, or syncope. Once these symptoms develop, the patient's average life expectancy is 2 to 3 years. The valve should be replaced and the left anterior descending artery bypassed before the patient develops an end-stage cardiomyopathy that will not respond to surgical intervention. (**Ref. 1,** p. 2013; **Ref. 3,** p. 872)

32. (E) This patient represents significant mitral valve regurgitation. He has evidence of depressed left ventricular function. Being a class III, New York Heart Association (NYHA), operation should be very strongly considered because results of mitral valve repair/replacement in class IV patients are very poor. In general, individuals over the age of 40 to 45 should have coronary arteriography to rule out significant coronary artery disease that may need concomitant correction. (**Ref. 1,** pp. 2032–2035)

33. (A) Aspiration of septic material from the mouth or oropharynx is the most common cause leading to a lung abscess. Such aspiration might occur in unconscious patients during induction of anesthesia or even during sleep when postnasal discharge may be aspirated. (**Ref. 1,** p. 1709; **Ref. 2,** p. 984; **Ref. 3,** p. 722)

34. (D) The most common sites for lung abscess are the superior and posterior segments of the right lung. The right bronchus is in more direct continuity with the trachea, and hence, aspirated material is likely to enter the right bronchus. The superior and posterior segments are the most dependent ones in the supine position, and aspirated material is likely to gravitate to these segments. (**Ref. 1,** p. 1710; **Ref. 2,** p. 984; **Ref. 3,** p. 722)

35. (B) Insertion of a chest tube to drain the hemothorax is the best method of treating hemothorax of 500 cc or more. Needle aspiration is inadequate to empty the blood, and a chest tube is necessary. Most bleeding into the pleural cavity spontaneously ceases, and thoracotomy is not necessary. Transfusion of blood is only required when there is systemic evidence of hypovolemia. (**Ref. 1,** p. 263; **Ref. 3,** p. 681)

36. (A) Empyema is most frequently a postpneumonic process that can manifest as lobar pneumonia, pneumonitis, or lung abscess.

Infection spreads to the pleural space either directly, by lymphatics, or by hematogenous routes. (**Ref. 1,** p. 1724; **Ref. 2,** p. 990; **Ref. 3,** p. 676)

37. **(D)**   Resection has no place in the treatment of a fresh tuberculous lesion prior to drug therapy. Surgery in tuberculous disease of the lung is usually performed for chronic lesions after chemotherapy has brought the disease under control. Other indications for surgical intervention include massive life-threatening hemoptysis, bronchopleural fistula, and a mass lesion when carcinoma cannot be otherwise excluded. (**Ref. 1,** pp. 1734–1735; **Ref. 2,** pp. 996–997; **Ref. 3,** pp. 716–717)

38. **(D)**   In many instances of chronic constrictive pericarditis, calcification of the pericardium is seen on chest x-ray and is often the first clue to the diagnosis. (**Ref. 1,** p. 1819; **Ref. 2,** p. 1051; **Ref. 3,** p. 895)

39. **(C)**   The normal shunt, in the presence of patent ductus arteriosus, is left-to-right; in the presence of a right-to-left shunt, one should suspect other pathology in the heart or advanced pulmonary sclerosis. These are contraindications for surgery in patients with PDA. (**Ref. 1,** p. 1957; **Ref. 2,** p. 1062; **Ref. 3,** p. 810)

40. **(B)**   Long, narrow fingers are a feature of Marfan's syndrome and are not seen in tetralogy. Tetralogy of Fallot is a form of cyanotic heart disease, and clubbing of the fingers is present. All others are also features of tetralogy of Fallot. (**Ref. 1,** p. 1191; **Ref. 2,** p. 1090)

41. **(B)**   Trauma is a very infrequent cause of aneurysm of the ascending aorta. Most are due to degenerative connective tissue disease of the aortic media. Other causes are atherosclerosis, cystic medial degeneration, myxomatous degeneration, dissection, and infection. (**Ref. 1,** p. 1556; **Ref. 3,** p. 910)

42. **(B)**   Aneurysms of the ascending aorta produce a dilatation of the aortic ring and resulting aortic insufficiency. Rarely, the enlarged aorta causes superior vena caval syndrome. (**Ref. 1,** p. 1557; **Ref. 3,** pp. 910–911)

244 / Cardiothoracic Surgery

43. (B) Pleural mesotheliomas are frequently found in patients suffering from asbestosis. (**Ref. 1,** p. 1725; **Ref. 2,** p. 991)

44. (B) Patients with atrial septal defect have a left-to-right shunt with blood flow across the septal defect. However, the murmur is not from this area of the heart but rather is a systolic flow murmur due to increased blood flow through the pulmonic valve. The first heart sound is often accentuated, but most characteristic of this defect is that the second heart sound is split in all phases of respiration, resulting from increased right ventricular filling and prolonged emptying. (**Ref. 1,** p. 1880; **Ref. 2,** p. 1080; **Ref. 3,** p. 797)

45. (C) Patients with patent ductus arteriosus have a characteristic murmur that is continuous and rumbling. It is heard over the right second to third intercostal spaces and is often referred to as a "machinery" murmur. (**Ref. 1,** p. 1856; **Ref. 2,** p. 1062; **Ref. 3,** pp. 808–809)

46. (A) Ventricular septal defects are one of the most common congenital defects. Because the systolic pressure generated in the left ventricle is much higher than in the right ventricle, there is a left-to-right shunt. These patients have a loud, harsh, systolic murmur present over the third to fifth left intercostal spaces. There is generally also an associated thrill. (**Ref. 1,** p. 1902; **Ref. 2,** p. 1087)

47. (D) Patients with tetralogy of Fallot usually have a harsh systolic murmur audible over the pulmonary area and along the left sternal border. (**Ref. 1,** p. 1911; **Ref. 2,** p. 1090, **Ref. 3,** p. 814)

48. (B) Coccidioidomycosis is often associated with the presence of thin-walled cavities and pus in the lungs. (**Ref. 1,** p. 1714; **Ref. 3,** p. 722)

49. (C) North American blastomycosis produces skin lesions in addition to the pulmonary lesion. (**Ref. 1,** p. 1714; **Ref. 2,** p. 985; **Ref. 3,** p. 735)

50. (D) The lung cavity in cases of aspergillosis contains a fungus ball. (**Ref. 1,** p. 1715; **Ref. 2,** pp. 986–987; **Ref. 3,** p. 735)

51. **(A)** Histoplasmosis is the most frequent granulomatous lesion that produces a solitary lung nodule. (**Ref. 1,** pp. 1712–1713; **Ref. 2,** p. 985; **Ref. 3,** p. 719)

52. **(B)** Thymomas are the most frequent lesion in the superior mediastinum and are confined to this part of the mediastinum. (**Ref. 1,** p. 1776; **Ref. 2,** p. 1038; **Ref. 3,** pp. 760–761)

53. **(A)** Teratomas usually present in the anterior mediastinum. (**Ref. 1,** p. 1776; **Ref. 2,** p. 1030; **Ref. 3,** p. 761)

54. **(D)** Pericardial cysts are located in the middle mediastinum. (**Ref. 1,** p. 1776; **Ref. 2,** p. 1034; **Ref. 3,** p. 761).

55. **(C)** Neurogenic tumors are most common in the posterior mediastinum. (**Ref. 1,** p. 1776; **Ref. 2,** p. 1027; **Ref. 3,** p. 759)

56. **(C)** The probability of a solitary nodule being a carcinoma lesion increases with age. In the 60- to 69-year-old age range, the chance of malignancy is in excess of 50%. When faced with a nodular density on chest x-ray, it is useful to review previous films. If the same lesion had been present 2 or more years earlier and remains unchanged, the probability of its being a malignant tumor would be quite small. (**Ref. 1,** p. 1755)

57. **(C)** The normal range for $Paco_2$ lies between 38 and 42 torr. Values greater than 43 torr indicate hypoventilation and are indicative of severe pulmonary disease. A value of 50 torr would usually make this patient inoperable for any pulmonary resection. With increased age, there is a decrease in the arterial PO_2. The normal Pao_2 for a 60-year-old patient would be 81 torr. A value of 70 mm Hg would be lower than expected; however, it would not preclude a surgical resection. An FEV_1 of 1.5 liters would probably preclude pneumonectomy, but he could likely tolerate a lobectomy. In borderline cases, a ventilation/perfusion scan can be very helpful to determine percentage of function for the various areas of the lung. A right adrenal mass would be very worrisome. However, a lesion of this size, without other evidence of

metastatic disease, would have a low probability for being a metastatic lesion. This lesion should be evaluated prior to any surgical intervention using percutaneous, CT-directed biopsy. Enlarged mediastinal lymph nodes would be of considerable concern; however, a lymph node of this size would most likely not represent tumor. The paratracheal lymph nodes should be assessed prior to any resection by mediastinoscopy. A lymph node that is positive for tumor on the contralateral side would preclude resection. Extensive tumor involvement on the ipsilateral side would also preclude resection. (**Ref. 1,** pp. 1686–1689, 1750–1751)

58. **(D)**   This patient is rapidly developing respiratory failure. A respiratory rate greater than 40 breaths per minute and a Pao_2 less than 60 torr are indications for intubation and mechanical ventilation if the situation cannot be quickly corrected. In addition to the flail chest, this patient had evidence of pulmonary contusion. The latter may be a greater cause of respiratory insufficiency than the paradoxical movement of the flail segment, because it produces a ventilation/perfusion mismatch or shunt. Infusions of large volumes of fluid may increase the edema in the area of lung contusion and worsen the shunt. Narcotics may improve the pain, but will not improve the shunt and could further impair the patient respiratory efforts. Increasing the Fio_2 to 100% by face mask will do little to improve his oxygenation. (**Ref. 1,** p. 261; **Ref. 3,** p. 653)

59. **(A)**   The most common major congenital deformity of the sternum is pectus excavatum. The pectus can vary from a very mild defect to one that is quite severe with concomitant physiologic impairment—respiratory and cardiac insufficiency, especially during exercise. Poor self-image is often present in many of these patients. Surgical repair can give excellent results with very few complications. (**Ref. 1,** pp. 1761–1763; **Ref. 3,** p. 686)

60. **(C)**   Mediastinitis following cardiac procedures generally has a low incidence (1% to 2%). There are several factors that can increase the risk for certain patients groups. Obesity and diabetes increase infection rate in general, as does a bypass time of more

than three hours. Low flow states may cause decreased local host resistance to bacteria, and as many as half the patients with mediastinitis have had "low flow" phenomena. Even though this patient does not exhibit sternal wound drainage or an unstable sternum, infection beneath the sternum is still a high probability. Aspiration of the sternum or computed tomography looking for air/fluid levels can be helpful diagnostic tests. (**Ref. 1,** pp. 1796–1798)

12

Peripheral Vascular Surgery

W. Kirt Nichols
Michael Kikta

DIRECTIONS (Questions 1 through 13): Each of the questions or incomplete statements below is followed by five suggested answers or completions. Select the ONE that is best in each case.

---

1. Postthrombotic varicose veins are due to
   A. incompetent communicating veins
   B. destruction of deep veins
   C. destruction of superficial veins
   D. iliofemoral incompetence
   E. block of the long saphenous vein

2. Deep venous thrombosis prophylaxis is appropriate for all of the following patients EXCEPT
   A. a 67-year-old male undergoing a colectomy
   B. a 21-year-old male undergoing an outpatient open inguinal hernia repair
   C. a 21-year-old male in the ICU, comatose, with a closed head injury

D. a 60-year-old female undergoing open reduction and internal fixation (ORIF) of a hip fracture

E. a 53-year-old female undergoing resection of a lung carcinoma

3. Primary treatment of pulmonary embolism (PE) consists of
   A. anticoagulation
   B. inferior vena caval ligation
   C. thrombectomy
   D. pulmonary embolectomy
   E. antiplatelet agents

4. All the following are true in the case of a splenic artery aneurysm EXCEPT
   A. it is the least common visceral arterial aneurysm
   B. usually it is due to medial degeneration of the arterial wall
   C. it produces pain in the left hypochondrium radiating to the left shoulder
   D. plain x-ray may show a calcific ring of the aneurysm
   E. risk of rupture is high during pregnancy

5. In atherosclerotic stenosis of the internal carotid artery, the treatment of choice is
   A. thromboendarterectomy
   B. excision and end-to-end anastomosis
   C. bypass grafting
   D. ligation of the internal carotid artery
   E. antiplatelet agent

6. Nutritional changes resulting from chronic ischemia include all the following EXCEPT
   A. loss of hair
   B. brittle, opaque nails
   C. atrophy of the skin
   D. atrophy of the muscles
   E. osteoporosis

7. The MOST common site at which arterial emboli lodge is the
   A. aortic bifurcation
   B. common iliac bifurcation
   C. common femoral bifurcation
   D. cerebral circulation
   E. popliteal artery

8. A 35-year-old diabetic man presents in ketoacidosis with fever, leukocytosis, and pain in his left foot. Examination shows a swollen, red foot with marked dorsal swelling and an ulcer with foul-smelling drainage over the exposed, eroded first metatarsal head. Posterior tibial pulse is normal. There is marked tenderness over the arch of the foot. Which of the following statements about this man's therapy is correct?
   A. single drug antibiotic therapy with nafcillin should be instituted for gram-positive cellulitis
   B. immediate open transmetatarsal amputation is required
   C. incision and drainage of the dorsal foot abscess is required
   D. metatarsal resection, plantar incision, and drainage and broad-spectrum antibiotic coverage is required
   E. antibiotics, elevation, and hyperbaric oxygen are basic elements of therapy for this man

9. All of the following statements can be made regarding major amputations of the lower extremity EXCEPT
   A. above-the-knee amputations have a higher rate of healing than below-the-knee amputations
   B. patients with below-the-knee amputations are more likely to be rehabilitated with a prosthesis than those with above-the-knee amputations
   C. a knee disarticulation is preferable to a long above-the-knee amputation because it permits an end-bearing stump in ambulatory patients and provides greater ease of transfers in non-ambulatory patients
   D. below-the-knee amputees (BKA) expend about half as much energy to ambulate as do above-the-knee amputees (AKA)
   E. the recommended amputation for a nonambulatory patient with a knee contracture and dry gangrene of the foot is a below-the-knee amputation

10. The clinical features of thoracic outlet syndrome include all the following EXCEPT
    A. paresthesia along the ulnar border
    B. atrophy or wasting of the thenar eminence
    C. pain in the neck and shoulder
    D. diminished radial pulse on arm elevation
    E. ischemic gangrene of the digits

11. The MOST frequent site of disease in occlusive cerebrovascular disease is the
    A. middle cerebral artery
    B. carotid bifurcation
    C. basilar artery
    D. vertebral artery at its origin
    E. origin of the common carotid

12. The MOST frequent site for atherosclerotic aneurysms in the periphery is the
    A. carotid
    B. subclavian
    C. femoral
    D. popliteal
    E. ulnar

13. Popliteal artery aneurysms present frequently with
    A. rupture
    B. pain and tenderness
    C. mass
    D. ischemic symptoms caused by embolization
    E. effusion into the knee joint

DIRECTIONS (Questions 14 through 21): This section consists of a clinical situation followed by a series of questions. Study the situation and select the ONE best answer to each question following it.

Questions 14 through 17

A 70-year-old man is brought to the emergency room with a 4-hour history of severe low back and abdominal pain. He has a history of hypertension, treated with a beta blocker. Examination shows a thin, alert, oriented male. The heart rate is 80/min, and BP is 90/60 mm Hg. There is an 8-cm tender, pulsatile, midepigastric mass present. Pedal pulses are 1+, bilaterally.

14. Appropriate *initial* treatment includes all of the following EXCEPT
  A. placement of large-bore IV catheters and initiation of lactated Ringer's infusion
  B. send blood for type and cross, complete blood count (CBC), electrolytes, and coagulation profile
  C. CT scan of abdomen
  D. placement of a Foley catheter
  E. stat chest x-ray and ECG

15. After completion of the above treatments, the MOST appropriate procedure should be
  A. urgent aortogram and runoff study
  B. emergent laparotomy
  C. CT of abdomen and pelvis with IV and GI contrast administration
  D. peritoneal lavage
  E. abdominal ultrasound

16. Three days after undergoing an aortofemoral bypass, the patient developed melena and loose stools. The MOST likely cause of the problem is
  A. stress ulcer bleeding
  B. ulcerative colitis
  C. ischemic colitis
  D. aortoduodenal fistula
  E. disseminated intravenous coagulation (DIC) due to blood transfusion

17. Eighteen hours after an acute traumatic occlusion of the femoral artery, the patient was operated on, and arterial repair was performed. In the recovery room, it was noted that the calf on the injured side was hard and extremely tender. The MOST likely cause is
   A. undiagnosed venous injury
   B. reaction to revascularization
   C. unsuspected fracture in the leg
   D. compartment syndrome
   E. muscle spasm due to nerve injury

Questions 18 and 19

An elderly male presented with a pulsatile abdominal mass. An abdominal angiogram was obtained (Figure 12.1).

18. The process shown is
   A. infrarenal aortic occlusion
   B. a large vascular left renal tumor
   C. arteriovenous (AV) malformation in liver
   D. abdominal aortic aneurysm
   E. aneurysm of left common iliac artery with occlusion of right

19. The ideal treatment of this lesion is
   A. periodic observation
   B. aortic endarterectomy
   C. aortofemoral bypass
   D. axillofemoral bypass
   E. left nephrectomy

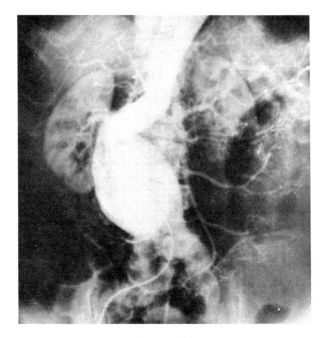

Figure 12.1

Questions 20 and 21

A 70-year-old male in cardiac failure presented with sudden onset of pain and coolness in the left arm of 12-hour duration. An angiogram of the left arm is shown in Figure 12.2.

20. The cause of the pain in the arm is
  A. thrombosis to the axillary artery
  B. embolization to the axillary artery
  C. axillary aneurysm with occlusion
  D. thromboangiitis obliterans
  E. Raynaud's disease

21. The treatment of the lesion shown in Figure 12.2 is
  A. heparinization alone
  B. heparinization and embolectomy
  C. thrombectomy

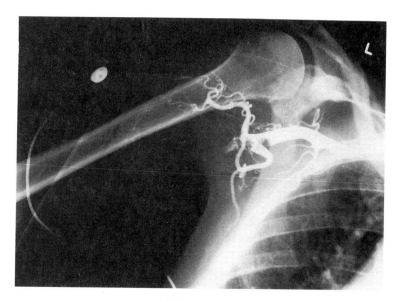

Figure 12.2

D. carotid–subclavian bypass
E. sympathectomy

DIRECTIONS (Questions 22 and 23): Each of the questions or incomplete statements below is followed by five suggested answers or completions. Select the ONE that is best in each case.

---

22. Techniques for diagnosis of deep venous thrombosis include all of the following EXCEPT
    A. phlebography
    B. radiofibrinogen studies
    C. ultrasonic studies
    D. venous flow rate studies
    E. electrical impedance test

23. A 45-year-old female complains of aching pain of the left upper arm that is aggravated after use of the arm. On using the arm for a long time, she also experiences dizziness and passes out. Examination reveals differences in the volume and tension of the pulses of the two upper limbs, and blood pressure is low in the left arm. The MOST likely pathology of this condition is

    A. coronary arteriosclerosis

    B. occlusion of the left subclavian artery proximal to the vertebral artery

    C. hypoplasia of the left radial artery

    D. cervical rib

    E. cervical disk prolapse

DIRECTIONS (Questions 24 through 49): This section consists of a clinical situation followed by a series of questions. Study the situation and select the ONE best answer to each question following it.

Questions 24 and 25

A 28-year-old white male is transferred to the emergency room 3 hours after being pushed down a flight of stairs in a brawl. He complains of pain in his left knee and numbness of his left leg. Examination shows a swollen left knee with a positive anterior drawer sign. He is unable to wiggle his toes and has numbness in the first dorsal web space. The foot is cool and pale. Pulses are not palpable, and there is no Doppler flow at the ankle.

24. All of the following diagnoses may be made in the above patient EXCEPT

    A. popliteal vein thrombosis

    B. peroneal nerve palsy

    C. popliteal artery thrombosis

    D. history of posterior knee dislocation

    E. acute arterial insufficiency

25. Optimal management of the injury should include

    A. complete ligamentous repair of the knee

    B. thrombectomy of the popliteal artery

    C. urgent direct repair of the popliteal artery, stabilization of the knee, and fasciotomy

    D. fasciotomy alone

    E. intra-arterial thrombolytic therapy and knee splinting

26. Regarding segmental femoropopliteal occlusive arterial disease, which of the following statements is true?

    A. the most common site is the superficial femoral artery within the adductor canal

    B. ulceration and gangrene are common

    C. the majority of patients are diabetic

    D. the rate of progression of disease is rapid

    E. patients are usually asymptomatic

Questions 27 and 28

A 57-year-old man returns to his room following a cardiac catheterization study through the left brachial artery at the elbow. You are called by the nurse 1 hour after the study because of an inability to find pulses at the wrist on that side. Examination confirms absent pulses, and the hand is cool to touch. The patient has paresthesias in the fingers and hand.

27. The MOST likely diagnosis is

    A. diminished cardiac output

    B. thrombosis of the brachial artery

    C. atheroembolism of the digital arteries

    D. vasospasm

    E. median nerve injury

28. Appropriate definitive management would be

    A. intravenous thrombolytic therapy

    B. anticoagulation with heparin

    C. continued observation and pulse checks

    D. early exploration and vascular repair

    E. vasodilator therapy

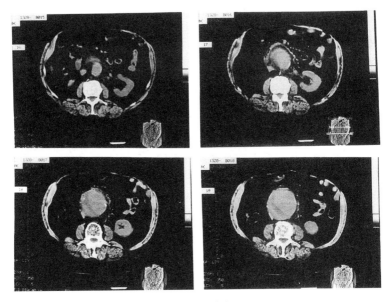

Figure 12.3

Questions 29 and 30

You were called to see a 69-year-old male who has been hospitalized for 2 days because of abdominal and flank pain. His hemoglobin has dropped from 13 g/dL to 10 g/dL. The vital signs include a blood pressure of 130/70 mm Hg and a heart rate of 80/min. He is obese with midabdominal tenderness. Representative images from a CT scan are shown in Figure 12.3.

29. Appropriate management of this man's problem includes
   A. aortogram with runoff
   B. cardiac catheterization
   C. urgent operation
   D. pulmonary function testing
   E. persantine thallium myocardial perfusion scan

30. The appropriate operation for this man is
   A. ligation of splenic artery aneurysm
   B. aneurysm resection and bypass

    C. axillobifemoral bypass

    D. sigmoid colectomy with end colostomy/Hartmann's procedure

    E. nephrolithotomy

Questions 31 through 35

A 68-year-old man presents to the hospital with acute onset of pain in his left lower extremity below the knee of 8 hours' duration. Examination shows a palpable pulse in the groin but absent pulses below this level. The foot is cool and pale, with diminished sensation but intact motor function.

31. The differential diagnosis may include all of the following EXCEPT

    A. arterial embolus

    B. hypovolemia

    C. thrombosis of a popliteal aneurysm

    D. acute arterial thrombosis at the site of a preexisting atherosclerotic narrowing

    E. traumatic arterial injury

32. The MOST sensitive tissue to acute hypoxemia secondary to acute peripheral arterial occlusion is

    A. peripheral nerve

    B. skin

    C. bone

    D. subcutaneous tissue

    E. nails and hair

33. Initial diagnostic procedures may include all of the following EXCEPT

    A. noninvasive doppler studies

    B. angiography

    C. complete physical examination

    D. nerve conduction velocities

    E. echocardiogram

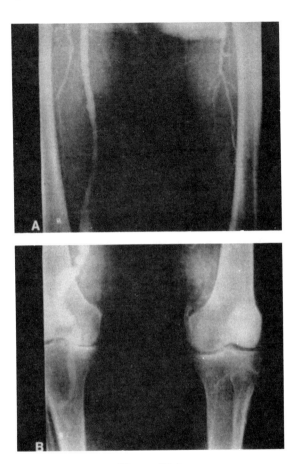

Figure 12.4

34. The angiogram shown in Figure 12.4, was obtained. The MOST likely cause of the left leg pain is
    A. popliteal aneurysm with acute thrombosis
    B. thrombosis of the superficial femoral artery
    C. thromboangiitis obliterans
    D. embolus to the popliteal artery
    E. ruptured Baker's cyst

35. Appropriate treatment for the lesions shown is
   A. anticoagulation with heparin
   B. embolectomy
   C. bypass of popliteal artery with autogenous saphenous vein
   D. amputation
   E. percutaneous balloon angioplasty

Question 36 through 39

Six hours following appropriate treatment, you are summoned to the patient's bedside. The nurse reports decreased motor and sensory function in the left leg and diminished pulsations at the ankle. Examination shows firm calf muscles with tenderness to palpation.

36. The MOST likely explanation is
   A. deep venous thrombosis
   B. occlusion of revascularized segment
   C. traumatic nerve injury
   D. compartment syndrome
   E. causalgia

37. The MOST appropriate management is
   A. heparin anticoagulation
   B. thrombolytic therapy
   C. reexploration and thrombectomy
   D. elevation and continued observation
   E. fasciotomy

38. After completion of the appropriate treatment, the nurse reports a decreased urine output. The urine in the collection tubing is red. The MOST likely explanation is
   A. hemorrhagic cystitis
   B. myoglobinuria
   C. hypovolemia
   D. anesthetic nephrotoxicity
   E. porphyria

39. Appropriate treatment would include all of the following EXCEPT
    A. acidifying the urine
    B. intravenous fluids
    C. mannitol
    D. alkalinizing the urine
    E. dextran

Questions 40 through 45

A 37-year-old female presents with hypertension and an abdominal bruit. An angiogram was obtained (see Figure 12.5).

40. The process which BEST explains her hypertension is
    A. fibromuscular dysplasia
    B. embolism to the renal artery

Figure 12.5

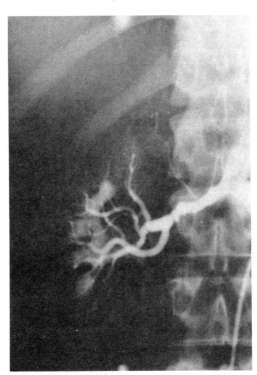

    C. renal artery aneurysm
    D. essential hypertension
    E. atherosclerotic renal artery stenosis

41. Proper evaluation should include all of the following EXCEPT
    A. radioisotopic renogram
    B. renin vein renin studies
    C. urinalysis
    D. serum creatinine
    E. serum electrolytes

42. Appropriate correction of the lesion shown might include
    A. nephrectomy
    B. aortofemoral bypass grafting
    C. percutaneous transluminal angioplasty
    D. endarterectomy
    E. lumbar sympathectomy

43. The pathophysiologic mechanism for this woman's hypertension is
    A. hypereninemia
    B. hypervolemia
    C. atherosclerosis
    D. sympathetic hyperactivity
    E. hypoaldosteronism

44. The definitive diagnosis of PE is best made by
    A. ventilation perfusion (VQ) scan
    B. chest x-ray
    C. depression of arterial O_2
    D. pulmonary angiogram
    E. duplex scan

45. Deep venous thrombosis is MOST definitively diagnosed by
    A. I^{121} fibrinogen scan
    B. CT scan
    C. venogram
    D. indium-labeled white cell scan
    E. Doppler ultrasonography

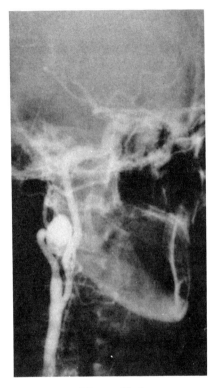

Figure 12.6

Questions 46 and 47

A 39-year-old woman complains of pain behind the right ear. In addition, she has experienced transient dizziness. Physical examination shows a slight fullness in the right neck. A bruit is noted over the carotid bifurcation. Her angiogram is shown Figure 12.6.

46. The process shown is
  A. carotid body tumor
  B. cervical lymphadenopathy
  C. branchial cleft cyst
  D. carotid aneurysm
  E. tortuosity of the subclavian artery

47. After appropriate treatment, the patient experiences drooping of the corner of the mouth on the right side. The best explanation is

  A. hypoglossal nerve injury
  B. ramus mandibularis nerve injury
  C. vagus nerve injury
  D. cerebrovascular accident (CVA)
  E. spinal accessory nerve injury

Questions 48 and 49

A 30-year-old woman seeks your advice regarding pain and paresthesia in the left hand, especially in the fourth and fifth fingers. In addition, she complains of fatigue and aching in the left shoulder.

48. Differential diagnosis includes all of the following EXCEPT

  A. cervical disk disease
  B. thoracic outlet syndrome
  C. cord tumor
  D. angina pectoris
  E. transient ischemic attacks

49. X-rays of the above patient are obtained and appear in Figure 12.7. They show an anatomic abnormality that may explain the patient's problem. The abnormality shown is

  A. a cervical rib
  B. a fractured clavicle
  C. a pneumothorax
  D. a cervical disk
  E. a spinal cord tumor

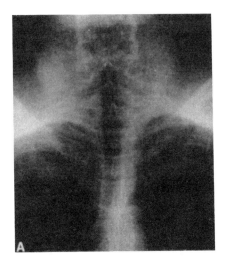

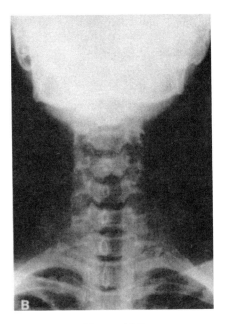

Figure 12.7

DIRECTIONS (Questions 50 through 72): Each group of questions below consists of lettered headings followed by a list of numbered words, phrases, or statements. For each numbered word, phrase, or statement, select the ONE lettered heading that is most closely associated with it. Each lettered heading may be used once, more than once, or not at all.

Questions 50 through 54

  A. metatarsal head ulcer
  B. supramalleolar ankle ulcer
  C. "punched out" anterior tibial area ulcer
  D. heel ulcer
  E. toe ulcer

50. Venous ulcer

51. Ulcer due to arterial insufficiency

52. Neurotropic, "malperforans" ulcer associated with diabetes mellitus

53. Usually a decubitus ulcer, may or may not be associated with arterial insufficiency

54. Poorly fitting shoes

Questions 55 through 59

  A. pentoxifylline
  B. urokinase
  C. heparin
  D. coumadin
  E. aspirin

55. Tissue plasminogen activator

56. Factors II, VII, IX, X; proteins C and S

57. Irreversible inhibitor of cyclooxygenase

58. Antithrombin III

59. Decreased blood viscosity

Questions 60 through 62

    A. balloon angioplasty (PTA)
    B. femoropopliteal bypass
    C. endarterectomy
    D. exercise program
    E. aortofemoral bypass

60. 75-year-old man with a 1-cm-long tight common iliac artery stenosis and one block claudication

61. 60-year-old man with an ischemic toe ulcer and a 20-cm-long occlusion of the superficial femoral artery

62. 55-year-old male smoker who drives a truck for a living and has half-mile calf claudication

Questions 63 through 67

    A. primary lymphedema
    B. secondary lymphedema
    C. chronic venous insufficiency
    D. renal failure or congestive heart failure
    E. arteriovenous (AV) malformation

63. Bilateral pitting edema, improves with elevation

64. Unilateral leg swelling developing after a deep venous thrombosis (DVT)

65. Firm, rubbery, nonpitting edema developing in a 20-year-old female

66. Leg swelling after radiation therapy for anal carcinoma

67. Limb hypertrophy, varicose veins, and capillary nevus in a child

Questions 68 through 72

- **A.** superior mesenteric artery embolism
- **B.** nonocclusive mesenteric ischemia
- **C.** superior mesenteric artery thrombosis
- **D.** mesenteric venous thrombosis
- **E.** chronic mesenteric ischemia

68. Sudden onset of severe abdominal pain, loose stools, and minimal abdominal tenderness in a woman with atrial fibrillation

69. Insidious onset of progressive abdominal pain, emesis, diarrhea, acidosis, leukocytosis, abdominal distention, and tenderness in an elderly man with angina, claudication, and a history of stroke

70. Progressive abdominal pain, distention, and vomiting in an elderly, dehydrated, bedridden lady

71. Postprandial pain and weight loss in an elderly man

72. Progressive abdominal pain, tenderness, and distention with diarrhea and vomiting in a patient with congestive heart failure treated with digoxin

Peripheral Vascular Surgery

Answers and Comments

1. **(A)** Postthrombotic varicose veins usually are due to damage to the valves and consequent incompetent perforating veins. (**Ref. 1,** p. 1490; **Ref. 2,** p. 1005)

2. **(B)** All of the other patients are at increased risk for DVT and PE due to immobility, prolonged operation, malignancy, or the presence of a long bone fracture. Appropriate measures for DVT prophylaxis may include subcutaneous heparin administration, oral coumadin, and intermittent pneumatic leg compression. (**Ref. 2,** pp. 990–991)

3. **(A)** The primary treatment of pulmonary embolism consists of anticoagulation, which usually is done with intravenous heparin, followed by oral anticoagulation with warfarin derivatives. (**Ref. 1,** pp. 1507–1508; **Ref. 2,** p. 1001)

4. **(A)** Aneurysms of the splenic artery are the most common visceral arterial aneurysms. Rupture is more likely in women during late pregnancy. (**Ref. 1,** p. 1564; **Ref. 2,** p. 1504)

5. **(A)** The treatment of choice for atherosclerotic occlusion of the internal carotid artery is thromboendarterectomy. Ligation should

not be performed because of a high risk of cerebral damage. By-pass grafting does not provide any better results than thromboen-darterectomy. (**Ref. 1,** pp. 1582–1583; **Ref. 2,** p. 967)

6. **(E)** Chronic ischemia usually does not lead to osteoporosis. The earliest signs are loss of hair and atrophy of the skin. Where there is a longstanding ischemia, atrophy of the muscles occurs. (**Ref. 2,** p. 930)

7. **(C)** The most common site for lodgement of arterial emboli is the common femoral artery. (**Ref. 1,** p. 1504; **Ref. 2,** p. 945)

8. **(D)** The description is that of a neurotropic metatarsal head ul-cer with metatarsal head osteomyelitis and a plantar abscess. Broad-spectrum antibiotic coverage for gram-positive, gram-neg-ative, and anaerobic organisms, and aggressive surgical drainage and removal of the necrotic, infected tissue are required. Major amputation as the initial treatment is rarely required unless frank gangrene is present. (**Ref. 1,** p. 956)

9. **(E)** Knee contracture is a contraindication to below-the-knee amputation because a functional prosthesis cannot be fitted. These patients are nonambulatory, and pressure against the end of the stump from the continuously flexed knee joint predisposes them to stump ulcers. (**Ref. 2,** pp. 1968,1973,1975)

10. **(B)** Clinical features of the thoracic outlet syndrome include all except atrophy or wasting of the thenar eminence. The muscles of the thenar eminence are supplied by the median nerve, and the roots involved in the thoracic outlet syndrome are C8 and T1. These do not significantly affect the muscles of the thenar emi-nence. Wasting of hypothenar muscles may occur. (**Ref. 1,** p. 1758; **Ref. 2,** p. 971)

11. **(B)** The most frequent site of occlusion in cerebral vascular dis-ease is the carotid bifurcation. Usually, the plaque is situated on the internal carotid side of the bifurcation and extends from one to two cm along its length. (**Ref 2,** p. 964)

12. **(D)** The popliteal artery is the most frequently affected site of peripheral atherosclerotic aneurysms. This has been attributed to

the repeated movements it undergoes behind the knee joint. (**Ref. 2,** p. 941)

13. (**D**) Most of the presenting symptoms of popliteal artery aneurysms are due to emboli arising from the aneurysmal sac. These lodge distally and produce ischemic symptoms. (**Ref. 2,** p. 941)

14. (**C**) 15. (**B**) 16. (**C**) This man has a classic history for a ruptured abdominal aortic aneurysm (AAA). He is hypotensive; his heart rate is normal because his ability to become tachycardic is blunted by the beta blocker. Plans should be made for immediate operation. CT scanning and/or abdominal ultrasound may be helpful when the diagnosis is less clear and in stable, normotensive patients. Aortography is time consuming and does not reliably establish the diagnosis of a ruptured AAA. Ischemic colitis is a potential complication of aortic reconstruction. The cause of inadequate colonic blood supply is ligation of the inferior mesenteric artery in the presence of inadequate collateral circulation. (**Ref. 1,** pp. 1551–1552; **Ref. 2,** pp. 939–940)

17. (**D**) Compartment syndromes occur following restoration of flow to ischemic tissues. Edema of muscles increases tissue pressure, and the pressure results in obliteration of flow. The problem is more common after delayed revascularization and may require fasciotomy. (**Ref. 1,** p. 1619; **Ref. 2,** p. 981)

18. (**D**) The angiogram shows a large, classic abdominal aneurysm. When they are large, they may deflect to the left. The aortic bifurcation is beyond the field of x-ray. (**Ref. 1,** pp. 1550–1551; **Ref. 2,** p. 935)

19. (**C**) The standard treatment of aortic aneurysm is an aortofemoral or aortoiliac bypass. Aneurysms with a diameter greater than 5 cm should be operated on because of risk of rupture. (**Ref. 1,** pp. 1553–1554; **Ref. 2,** pp. 934, 938)

20. (**B**) The sharp cut-off of blood flow high in the arm indicates acute occlusion, probably due to embolism. The lack of preformed collateral indicates that it is not a chronic occlusive problem. There is no evidence of aneurysm; Raynaud's disease and

thromboangiitis do not produce a sudden sharp occlusion. (**Ref. 2,** pp. 945–947)

21. **(B)** The lesion is embolic, and the treatment is immediate heparinization and embolectomy. Heparinization alone is not sufficient. All other operations offer no benefit in acute embolic occlusion. (**Ref. 2,** p. 948)

22. **(D)** Venous flow rate studies are not of great value in the diagnosis of deep venous thrombosis and are not used in a clinical setting. Phlebography provides the absolute proof of deep venous thrombosis. There are reports that indicate that radiofibrinogen, ultrasonic methods, and electrical impedance studies provide useful clinical data. (**Ref. 2,** pp. 962–963)

23. **(B)** The diagnosis in this patient appears to be a subclavian steal syndrome. The pathology of the condition is an occlusion of the left subclavian artery proximal to the origin of the vertebral. The blood to the left subclavian artery flows from the opposite vertebral artery through the circle of Willis. Exercise causes a "steal" of blood from the vertebral artery into the distal subclavian, thereby depriving the brain of oxygenated blood. (**Ref. 1,** p. 1584; **Ref. 2,** p. 962)

24. **(A)** 25. **(C)** This man has sustained a popliteal artery injury from a posterior knee dislocation. He has acute arterial insufficiency from popliteal artery thrombosis due to stretching of the artery, resulting in intimal cracking and exposure of the underlying thrombogenic adventitia. The resultant neural ischemia produces peroneal nerve palsy. Acute repair with bypass of the injured segment or resection and interposition grafting of the injured segment is required. The knee must be stabilized, usually by external fixation. A calf fasciotomy will probably be necessary to prevent a postrevascularization compartment syndrome. Thrombolytic therapy may restore arterial patency but fails to address the injured artery, which would likely rethrombose unless repaired. (**Ref. 1,** pp. 1613, 1622; **Ref. 2,** pp. 943, 981)

26. **(A)** The most common site for segmental femoropopliteal occlusive disease is the superficial femoral artery within the adductor canal. Possibly the constant trauma resulting from the con-

tracting tendon may predispose this site. The presenting feature is usually claudication with exercise. Rest pain is not an early presentation. (**Ref. 2,** p. 953)

27. **(B)**   Catheter injury is a common mechanism that may lead to thrombosis. (**Ref. 1,** pp. 1618–1619; **Ref. 2,** p. 981)

28. **(D)**   Early operative repair minimizes the effects of ischemia and the development of late sequelae. (**Ref. 1,** p. 1619; **Ref. 2,** p. 981)

29. **(C)**   **30. (B)**   The CT scan shows blood in the retroperitoneum outside of a large abdominal aortic aneurysm, diagnostic of contained rupture of an abdominal aortic aneurysm. The differential diagnosis of a ruptured AAA includes many common causes of abdominal and back pain, often delaying the diagnosis in hemodynamically stable or obese patients. Once the diagnosis is made, plans should be made for urgent operation. Other diagnostic tests are not needed. Aneurysm resection and bypass is the preferred operation for AAA. Axillobifemoral bypass, an extracavitary operation, fails to treat the aneurysm. Kidney stones and diverticulitis, treatable by choices D and E, are often included in the differential diagnosis of ruptured AAA. (**Ref. 1,** pp. 1552–1553; **Ref. 2,** pp. 938–939)

31. **(B)**   All of the other diagnoses listed may produce arterial occlusion. History may be quite helpful. (**Ref. 2,** p. 942)

32. **(A)**   Nerve and skeletal muscle are exquisitely sensitive to hypoxemia. Paralysis and paresthesia are important warning signs. (**Ref. 2,** p. 943)

33. **(D)**   Nerve conduction velocities are not indicated in patients with acute arterial insufficiency. The other studies listed may identify the site or source of the occlusion. (**Ref. 2,** pp. 944–945)

34. **(A)**   The angiogram shows an occlusion in the left popliteal artery. The right popliteal artery shows a popliteal aneurysm. Since popliteal aneurysms are frequently bilateral, it is most likely the acute presentation is due to thrombosis of a left popliteal aneurysm. (**Ref. 2,** p. 942)

35. (C) Bypass is preferred prior to distal embolization and/or thrombosis, if possible. The saphenous vein is the graft of choice. (**Ref. 2,** p. 942)

36. (D) The firm calf muscles and diminished pulses and nerve function following restoration of flow after prolonged ischemia suggest a compartment syndrome. (**Ref. 1,** p. 1619; **Ref. 2,** p. 981)

37. (E) The appropriate treatment for a compartment syndrome is fasciotomy. (**Ref. 1,** p. 1619; **Ref. 2,** p. 981)

38. (B) Reperfusion of severely ischemic muscles may produce a washout of myoglobin, which may injure the kidney. (**Ref. 2,** p. 461)

39. (A) Appropriate treatment includes alkalinizing the urine and establishing a diuresis. (**Ref. 2,** p. 461)

40. (A) The corrugated or "string of beads" appearance is characteristic of fibromuscular dysplasia. (**Ref. 2,** p. 961)

41. (A) The radioisotopic renogram is associated with a high incidence of false-positive and false-negative results, which limits its usefulness. (**Ref. 2,** p. 962)

42. (C) Nephrectomy is useful only when the appropriate kidney is so damaged it does not contribute to total renal function and it acts as a pressor kidney. Endarterectomy is useful in atherosclerotic lesions only. *Early* results of percutaneous angioplasty appear comparable to surgical results. (**Ref. 2,** p. 963)

43. (A) Unilateral renal artery stenosis, comparable to the "two-kidney, one-clip" Goldblatt model of hypertension, produces hypertension through sustained hyperreninemia. (**Ref. 2,** pp. 961–962)

44. (D) A normal lung scan reliably rules out a PE. A high-probability lung scan can accurately make the diagnosis of a PE, but less than one-third of patients with a PE will have such a scan. Pulmonary arteriography is the most accurate test for diagnosis of a PE. (**Ref. 2,** p. 998)

45. (C) A good quality duplex ultrasonogram is 95% accurate for diagnosing DVT and is commonly used to make this diagnosis. Venography, however, is the "gold standard." (**Ref. 2,** p. 993)

46. (D) The angiogram shows a tortuous carotid artery with a saccular aneurysm above the bifurcation. (**Ref. 2,** p. 965)

47. (B) Many nerve palsies may occur after carotid artery surgery. The one described best fits the ramus mandibularis branch of VII. (**Ref. 2,** p. 968)

48. (E) The patient described has thoracic outlet syndrome with neural symptoms in the ulnar distribution. Differential diagnosis includes angina, cord tumors, and cervical disk disease. (**Ref. 2,** pp. 919, 971)

49. (A) The x-ray demonstrates the presence of a left cervical rib. (**Ref. 2,** p. 969)

50. (B) A typical ulcer due to chronic venous insufficiency develops around the malleolar, or gaiter, area. The medial malleolar area is most commonly affected. (**Ref. 2,** pp. 954, 1005)

51. (C) Ulcers due to arterial insufficiency typically occur in the anterior tibial area, lateral ankle area, or on the foot. They have a characteristic "punched out" appearance with sharp well-defined edges and poor granulation tissue in the ulcer base. (**Ref. 2,** p. 954)

52. (A) The malperforans or plantar ulcer over the metatarsal head, or malperforans ulcer, occurs in diabetics for two reasons. The sensory neuropathy of diabetes permits repeated trauma to the area because the foot is insensate. Diabetics also have atrophy of the intrinsic foot muscles, resulting in a high-arch foot deformity with increased prominence of the metatarsal heads. (**Ref. 2,** p. 956)

53. (D) Heel ulcers usually develop from prolonged pressure on the heel in bedridden patients. Arterial insufficiency may prevent healing of these ulcers, despite protective measures. (**Ref. 2,** p. 954)

54. **(E)** Rubbing of the sides or tips of the toes may cause ulcers in diabetics with sensory neuropathy or in patients with arterial insufficiency. (**Ref. 2,** pp. 954, 956–957)

55. **(B)** Urokinase is a direct activator of tissue plasminogen. (**Ref. 2,** pp. 928, 949)

56. **(D)** Coumadin inhibits the Vitamin K-dependent coagulation proteins. (**Ref. 2,** p. 928)

57. **(E)** Aspirin inhibits platelet action by irreversibly inhibiting platelet cyclooxygenase. (**Ref. 2,** p. 928)

58. **(C)** Heparin binds to and increases the activity of antithrombin III. (**Ref. 2,** p. 928)

59. **(A)** Pentoxifylline decreases blood viscosity and also inhibits platelet function. (**Ref. 2,** p. 954)

60. **(A)** Short iliac artery stenoses can be satisfactorily treated with PTA, with patency rates approaching those of operative procedures. (**Ref. 2,** p. 952)

61. **(B)** Bypass procedures are more durable than PTA for long occlusions of the superficial femoral artery. (**Ref. 2,** p. 955)

62. **(D)** This sedentary man with nondisabling calf claudication should first stop smoking and begin a structured exercise program before interventional therapy is considered. (**Ref. 2,** p. 954)

63. **(D)** Bilateral pitting edema is usually associated with renal failure, cardiac failure, and conditions causing hypoproteinemia, such as hepatic cirrhosis or malnutrition. (**Ref. 2,** p. 1011)

64. **(C)** Limb swelling after a DVT may be due to venous outflow obstruction or venous valvular insufficiency with reflux. (**Ref. 2,** p. 1005)

65. **(A)** Congenital distal lymphatic hypoplasia causes firm nonpitting edema. Most patients are women who develop symptoms shortly after puberty. (**Ref. 2,** p. 1011)

66. **(B)** Postradiation fibrosis of the lymphatic channels, malignant infiltration, chronic infection, and surgical lymphadenectomy are common causes of secondary lymphedema. (**Ref. 2,** p. 1011)

67. **(E)** Klippel–Trenaunay syndrome, a type of venous dysplasia that is an AV malformation, is a rare cause of leg swelling and limb length discrepancy in children. (**Ref. 2,** pp. 977, 1011)

68. **(A)** 69. **(C)** 70. **(D)** 71. **(E)** 72. **(B)** The typical characteristic of early acute intestinal ischemia is severe abdominal pain out of proportion to the degree of abdominal tenderness present. Gut emptying, manifested as emesis and diarrhea, is common. The clinical setting is a good guide to the pathology, although angiography and/or findings at laparotomy are diagnostic. Symptoms of chronic mesenteric ischemia may precede SMA or celiac thrombosis. (**Ref. 2,** pp. 958–959, 1495–1503)

13

Pediatric Surgery
Mary Alice Helikson
Patricia Barker

DIRECTIONS (Questions 1 through 56): Each of the questions or incomplete statements below is followed by five suggested answers or completions. Select the ONE that is best in each case.

1. Which of the following is LEAST important for thermoregulation in a premature newborn?
   A. nonshivering thermogenesis
   B. neutral thermal environment
   C. radiant warming device
   D. skin temperature monitoring
   E. hair and subcutaneous tissue

2. Normal hourly urinary output for a 22-pound infant is
   A. 15 mL
   B. 5 mL
   C. 20 mL
   D. 10 mL
   E. 22 mL

3. A safe and effective fluid bolus for a hypotensive child is
  A. 5 mL/kg normal saline
  B. 30 mL/kg one-fourth normal saline
  C. 20 mL/kg Ringer's lactate
  D. 40 mL/kg 5% dextrose water
  E. 10 mL/kg one-half normal saline

4. Which of the following is true of ALL infants with congenital intestinal obstruction?
  A. maternal polyhydramnios present
  B. nasogastric sump indicated
  C. bilious vomiting present
  D. infant fails to pass meconium
  E. abdominal distention present

5. Associated congenital anomalies are LEAST frequent with
  A. ileal atresia
  B. imperforate anus
  C. esophageal atresia
  D. omphalocele
  E. duodenal atresia

6. The initial diagnostic test for newborn who drools saliva is
  A. esophogram
  B. bronchoscopy
  C. upper GI series
  D. esophagoscopy
  E. nasogastric tube and chest x-ray

7. The major cause of death in infants with esophageal atresia is
  A. aspiration pneumonia
  B. diarrhea and dehydration
  C. anesthetic complications
  D. associated anomalies
  E. vomiting and malnutrition

8. Trisomy 21 is associated with all of the following EXCEPT
  A. Hirschsprung's disease
  B. duodenal atresia
  C. diaphragmatic hernia

   D. undescended testes

   E. congenital heart disease

9. The "double bubble" sign on newborn abdominal x-ray is diagnostic for

   A. incarcerated inguinal hernia

   B. duodenal atresia

   C. Meckel's diverticulum

   D. pyloric stenosis

   E. malrotation with volvulus

10. The primary etiology of jejunal and ileal atresias is

   A. vascular accident

   B. maternal drug abuse

   C. birth injury

   D. chromosomal anomaly

   E. maternal diabetes

11. All of the following refer to meconium ileus EXCEPT

   A. pancreatic enzyme deficiency

   B. often relieved with hypertonic enema

   C. hereditary disease

   D. affects lungs, pancreas and skin

   E. aganglionic distal intestine

12. Definitive neonatal diagnosis of Hirschsprung's disease is made by

   A. delayed stool production

   B. abdominal distention

   C. barium enema

   D. rectal suction biopsy

   E. abdominal x-rays

13. MOST full-term, healthy, newborn infants pass meconium by

   A. 12 hours of age

   B. 60 hours of age

   C. 24 hours of age

   D. 48 hours of age

   E. 36 hours of age

14. The MOST important exam in the work-up of imperforate anus is
   A.   thoracic and lumbosacral x-rays
   B.   perineal examination
   C.   echocardiography
   D.   renal ultrasound
   E.   passage of a nasogastric tube

15. Necrotizing enterocolitis is associated with all of the following EXCEPT
   A.   blood in the gastric aspirate
   B.   decreasing platelet count
   C.   abdominal distention
   D.   pneumatosis intestinalis
   E.   persistent metabolic acidosis

16. Definitive diagnosis of malrotation with midgut volvulus is made by
   A.   elective upper GI series
   B.   sudden onset of bilious vomiting
   C.   abdominal distention and tenderness
   D.   white blood count and differential
   E.   emergent barium enema

17. Which of the following conditions requires immediate surgery?
   A.   duodenal atresia
   B.   bacterial sepsis
   C.   jejunal atresia
   D.   midgut volvulus
   E.   duodenal stenosis

18. Treatment of abdominal wall defects includes all of the following EXCEPT
   A.   maintaining infant in thermal neutral zone
   B.   nasogastric sump decompression
   C.   resection of small intestine
   D.   intravenous fluid resuscitation
   E.   placing infant in bowel bag up to axillae

19. Symptoms and signs of diaphragmatic hernia include all of the following EXCEPT
    A. decreased breath sounds on left
    B. failure to pass meconium
    C. barrel chest and scaphoid abdomen
    D. respiratory distress and cyanosis
    E. heart sounds shifted to the right

20. All of the following may present with bilious vomiting EXCEPT
    A. pyloric stenosis
    B. duodenal atresia
    C. annular pancreas
    D. jejunal atresia
    E. midgut volvulus

21. Which of the following is associated with both omphalocele and gastroschisis?
    A. abdominal wall defect
    B. intestinal nonrotation
    C. prenatal diagnosis
    D. immediate surgical treatment required
    E. all of the above

22. Which of the following is the daily caloric requirement for a 4-kg neonate?
    A. 640 calories
    B. 320 calories
    C. 480 calories
    D. 560 calories
    E. 720 calories

23. All of the following congenital alimentary tract obstructions are associated with maternal polyhydramnios EXCEPT
    A. esophageal atresia without tracheoesophageal fistula
    B. high jejunal atresia
    C. pylonic atresia or antral web
    D. esophageal atresia with tracheoesophageal fistula
    E. duodenal atresia

24. Colon atresia is usually associated with all of the following EX-CEPT
   A. bilious vomiting within the first 24 hours of life
   B. prematurity
   C. soap bubble appearance of the atretic loop on abdominal x-ray
   D. abdominal distention
   E. right colon predominance

25. The MOST appropriate operative procedure for correction of a choledochal cyst is
   A. resection of the cyst and Roux-en-Y hepatojejunostomy
   B. cystoduodenostomy
   C. resection of the cyst and primary bile duct anastomosis
   D. cystojejunostomy
   E. resection of the cyst and choledochoduodenostomy

26. All of the following are associated with gastroesophageal reflux EXCEPT
   A. use of bronchodilators
   B. esophageal atresia
   C. neurologic impairment
   D. sudden infant death
   E. biliary atresia

27. Symptoms of gastroesophageal reflux include all of the following EXCEPT
   A. apnea and bradycardia
   B. failure to thrive
   C. hematemesis
   D. polyhydramnios
   E. recurrent pneumonia

28. The TRUE statement concerning the problem demonstrated in the barium enema shown in Figure 13.1 is
   A. it usually has a pathologic leadpoint
   B. it produces colonic obstruction
   C. it is often reduced by contrast enema
   D. it is more frequent in females
   E. it presents before 6 months of age

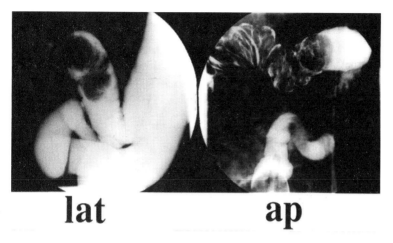

lat   ap

Figure 13.1

29. Reasons for neonatal umbilical discharge include all of the following EXCEPT
    A. patent urachus
    B. Meckel's diverticulum
    C. omphalomesenteric duct remnant
    D. umbilical granuloma
    E. urachal sinus

30. Diagnostic study for bleeding Meckel's diverticulum is
    A. technetium scan
    B. sigmoidoscopy
    C. small bowel series
    D. arteriography
    E. barium enema

31. All of the following are true of juvenile polyps EXCEPT
    A. most rectosigmoid
    B. autoamputation common
    C. usually solitary
    D. produce rectal bleeding
    E. often premalignant

32. All of the following are true of extrahepatic biliary atresia EXCEPT
   A. probably due to intrauterine viral infection
   B. hepatoportoenterostomy unsuccessful after 3 months of age
   C. improved outcome with early diagnosis
   D. presents with jaundice and right upper quadrant mass
   E. liver transplantation has improved survival

33. Evaluation of a jaundiced 1-month-old infant includes all of the following EXCEPT
   A. liver function battery
   B. hepatobiliary scan
   C. observation period
   D. operative cholangiogram
   E. abdominal ultrasound

34. Which of the following is true regarding appendicitis in a young child (versus adult)?
   A. patient not as dehydrated
   B. perforation more common
   C. history more helpful
   D. inversion appendectomy performed
   E. physical exam less important

35. All of the following may mimic appendicitis in a child EXCEPT
   A. acute renal failure
   B. viral gastroenteritis
   C. mittelschmerz
   D. Meckel's diverticulitis
   E. sickle cell crisis

36. Each of the following urine analysis findings is consistent with retrocecal appendicitis EXCEPT
   A. large ketones
   B. 5 WBC/hpf
   C. specific gravity 1.030
   D. 5 RBC/hpf
   E. many bacteria

37. All of the following are correct statements about hemangiomas EXCEPT
    A. they are common neoplasms of infancy
    B. most are treated with close observation
    C. spontaneous involution is frequent
    D. they are cavernous more frequently than capillary
    E. the majority occur on the head or neck

38. The MOST frequent organism associated with neck abscess in childhood is
    A. mononucleosis
    B. cat scratch
    C. *Staphylococcus aureus*
    D. mycobacteria
    E. histoplasmosis

39. Common neck masses in a young child include all of the following EXCEPT
    A. branchial remnant
    B. lymphoma
    C. cystic hygroma
    D. lymphadenitis
    E. thyroglossal remnant

40. Infant inguinal hernias are associated with all of the following EXCEPT
    A. delayed repair
    B. prematurity
    C. male sex
    D. incarceration
    E. right-sidedness

41. Incarcerated inguinal hernia is associated with all of the following EXCEPT
    A. ischemic testis
    B. intestinal gangrene
    C. small bowel obstruction
    D. premature birth
    E. infarcted ovary

42. All of the following phrases regarding undescended testes are true EXCEPT
   A. usually palpable
   B. prone to torsion
   C. associated with a hernia sac
   D. predisposed to malignancy
   E. usually bilateral

43. The ideal age for orchidopexy is
   A. 10 to 12 years
   B. 5 to 6 years
   C. 12 to 15 months
   D. 3 to 6 months
   E. at diagnosis

44. All of the following statements about umbilical hernias are correct EXCEPT
   A. low risk for incarceration
   B. defects >2 cm close spontaneously
   C. 80% involute by 4 years of age
   D. more common in females and blacks
   E. repair indicated before kindergarten

45. The chest x-ray of a child with foreign body aspiration may demonstrate
   A. mediastinal shift
   B. air trapping
   C. atelectasis
   D. normal chest
   E. any of the above

46. The MOST dangerous esophageal foreign body is
   A. toy part
   B. unchewed food
   C. quarter
   D. button battery
   E. safety pin

47. Physician responsibility for child abuse includes all of the following EXCEPT
    A. calling hotline number
    B. informing parents
    C. determining abuser
    D. treating injuries
    E. hospitalizing child

48. The injury LEAST suspicious for child abuse or neglect is
    A. immersion burn
    B. fractured spleen
    C. femur fracture in a 2-year-old
    D. perineal injury
    E. duodenal trauma

49. The primary cause of death in children 1 to 14 years of age is
    A. trauma
    B. congenital defects
    C. infectious diseases
    D. premature birth
    E. cancer

50. All of the following are correct statements about injured children EXCEPT
    A. gastric dilation is more common than in adults
    B. blood volume is smaller than in adults
    C. thermoregulation improves with age
    D. metabolic rate is higher than in adults
    E. penetrating trauma is more common than blunt

51. Which of the following is LEAST important in resuscitation of a pediatric trauma victim?
    A. secure vascular access
    B. adequate ventilation
    C. good oxygenation
    D. intravenous pressors
    E. fluid resuscitation

52. All of the following statements are true of pediatric trauma victims EXCEPT
   A. gastric dilatation produces acute pain
   B. computed tomography (CT) is very helpful
   C. peritoneal lavage is frequently indicated
   D. nonoperative management is common
   E. separation from parents is poorly tolerated

53. All of the following are true of Wilms' tumor EXCEPT
   A. may produce hypertension or hematuria
   B. majority diagnosed between 1 and 4 years of age
   C. cure rate over 80%
   D. associated with aniridia and hemihypertrophy
   E. survival not affected by histology

54. All of the following are true of neuroblastomas EXCEPT
   A. most diagnosed before 8 years of age
   B. may produce proptosis, black eyes, or nystagmus
   C. most secrete catecholamine byproducts
   D. majority present with localized disease
   E. tumor calcification common

55. The MOST common abdominal tumors in toddlers are
   A. Wilms' tumor and hepatoblastoma
   B. lymphoma and rhabdomyosarcoma
   C. neuroblastoma and Wilms' tumor
   D. hepatoblastoma and lymphoma
   E. rhabdomyosarcoma and neuroblastoma

56. Sacrococcygeal teratoma is associated with all of the following EXCEPT
   A. external or pelvic mass
   B. male predominance
   C. exsanguinating hemorrhage
   D. cesarean delivery
   E. malignant potential

DIRECTIONS (Questions 57 through 66): This section consists of a clinical situation followed by a series of questions. Study the situation and select the ONE best answer to each question following it.

Questions 57 through 59

A 3-week-old male presents with projectile vomiting void of bile. He appears to be hungry all the time and has lost weight since his 2-week checkup.

57. The MOST likely diagnosis is
A. duodenal stenosis
B. adrenogenital syndrome
C. aminoaciduria
D. gastroesophageal reflux
E. pyloric stenosis

58. The diagnostic physical finding in the above condition is
A. abdominal tenderness
B. peristaltic waves in lower abdomen
C. hyperactive bowel sounds
D. olive-shaped mass in upper abdomen
E. abdominal distention

59. If the physical exam is NOT diagnostic, which of the following tests should be obtained?
A. sweat chloride
B. esophageal pH probe
C. abdominal ultrasound
D. urine metabolic screen
E. abdominal films

Questions 60 through 63

A 9-month-old male is brought to the emergency room after passing blood and mucus per anus. There is an 18-hour history of intermittent severe abdominal colic associated with vomiting. Between attacks of pain the infant is lethargic.

60. The MOST likely diagnosis is
   A. peptic ulcer disease
   B. intussusception
   C. esophagitis
   D. juvenile polyps
   E. infectious diarrhea

61. Physical examination reveals all of the following EXCEPT
   A. absent bowel sounds
   B. empty right lower quadrant
   C. rectal blood
   D. epigastric sausage-shaped mass
   E. abdominal distention

62. Plain abdominal films are likely to show
   A. dilated stomach
   B. air-filled rectosigmoid
   C. nothing remarkable
   D. patchy small bowel air
   E. absent cecal air

63. The MOST important additional investigation is
   A. abdominal ultrasound
   B. upper GI series
   C. abdominal CT
   D. contrast enema
   E. small bowel series

Questions 64 through 66

An irritable 6-week-old boy is brought to urgent care clinic with a right groin mass. On past medical history, you find that he was born at 34 weeks' gestation and remained in the neonatal intensive care unit until 2 weeks ago.

64. The MOST likely diagnosis is
    A. noncommunicating hydrocele
    B. testicular torsion
    C. inguinal lymphadenitis
    D. communicating hydrocele
    E. incarcerated inguinal hernia

65. Which of the following is appropriate initial management?
    A. sustained gentle pressure aimed at reduction
    B. duplex Doppler scan
    C. intravenous antibiotics
    D. diagnostic aspiration
    E. incision and drainage

66. Possible complications include all of the following EXCEPT
    A. hypovolemic shock
    B. intestinal perforation
    C. infertility
    D. testicular atrophy
    E. intestinal obstruction

Pediatric Surgery

Answers and Comments

1. **(E)** Neonates are unable to shiver and have a large surface area with little subcutaneous tissue. External monitoring and warming devices help maintain a neutral thermal environment and minimize metabolic requirements. (**Ref. 1,** p. 1149; **Ref. 2,** p. 1683)

2. **(D)** The infant kidney does not produce concentrated urine but is able to handle fluid loads. A urinary volume of 1 mL/kg/hr, in the absence of diuretics, indicates adequate hydration. (**Ref. 1,** p. 1150; **Ref. 2,** p. 1682)

3. **(C)** Untreated hypotension in an infant or child rapidly progresses to cardiac arrest. Immediate infusion of 20 mL/kg of isotonic fluid (lactated Ringer's) returns vital signs toward normal. (**Ref. 1,** pp. 1151, 1175; **Ref. 2,** p. 1682)

4. **(B)** All are signs of congenital intestinal obstruction, but none is diagnostic or universal. All patients with intestinal obstruction benefit from efficient nasogastric decompression. (**Ref. 1,** pp. 1151–1152; **Ref. 2,** pp. 1695–1696)

5. **(A)** Esophageal atresia and anorectal malformation are part of the VACTERL association of anomalies. Duodenal atresia is associated with Down syndrome. A majority of infants with omphalocele have other congenital defects. Jejunal and ileal atresias

are infrequently associated with other anomalies. (**Ref. 1,** pp. 1152, 1154, 1162; **Ref. 2,** pp. 1690–1691)

6. (**E**)   Esophageal atresia with blind proximal pouch and distal tracheoesophageal fistula is present in 85% of infants with abnormal foregut division. Chest x-ray with nasogastric tube in place locates the end of the pouch, while air in the stomach documents the fistula. (**Ref. 1,** p. 1152; **Ref. 2,** pp. 1690–1691)

7. (**D**)   Severe associated defects and complications of prematurity are the most frequent causes of death in infants with esophageal atresia. Early diagnosis prevents, and critical care successfully treats, the pulmonary infections that historically plagued these infants. (**Ref. 1,** p. 1154; **Ref. 2,** p. 1691)

8. (**C**)   Duodenal atresia, endocardial cushion defects, Hirschsprung's disease, and cryptorchidism are more frequent in patients with Trisomy 21. Diaphragmatic hernia is not associated with a chromosomal anomaly. (**Ref. 1,** pp. 1154, 1158)

9. (**B**)   In a newborn with duodenal atresia, the two air bubbles on abdominal films are dilated stomach and duodenum. With pyloric stenosis, only the stomach is dilated. Plain films are not diagnostic for Meckel's diverticulum or midgut volvulus. Incarcerated inguinal hernia produces a distal small bowel obstruction. (**Ref. 1,** p. 1154)

10. (**A**)   Jejunal and ileal atresias result from intrauterine vascular accidents after the first trimester. About 10% are associated with cystic fibrosis. (**Ref. 1,** p. 1155; **Ref. 2,** p. 1696)

11. (**E**)   Meconium ileus is a manifestation of cystic fibrosis. Hypertonic contrast enema is diagnostic and is often therapeutic in uncomplicated cases. Aganglionic distal bowel is characteristic of Hirschsprung's disease. (**Ref. 1,** p. 1156; **Ref. 2,** pp. 1698, 1702)

12. (**D**)   The pathology of Hirschsprung's disease is absence of ganglion cells in the distal colon. Diagnosis is established by submucosal suction biopsy of the rectum. (**Ref. 1,** p. 1158; **Ref. 2,** p. 1702)

13. (C) Almost all healthy term infants pass meconium within 24 hours of birth. Delayed passage of meconium is the cardinal early symptom of Hirschsprung's disease. (**Ref. 1,** p. 1158; **Ref. 2,** p. 1702)

14. (B) Over 85% of infants with anorectal malformations have an associated fistulous tract, often visible on thorough perineal exam. The other examinations detect anomalies of the VACTERL association. (**Ref. 1,** p. 1159; **Ref. 2,** p. 1703)

15. (A) All are typical of necrotizing enterocolitis except upper gastrointestinal bleeding. Occult or gross rectal bleeding is a common finding in affected infants. (**Ref. 1,** p. 1160; **Ref. 2,** p. 1700)

16. (E) Bilious vomiting is an early symptom of midgut volvulus. Positive physical examination and laboratory findings occur late. Upper and lower contrast studies are diagnostic. Treatment delay results in midgut infarction. (**Ref. 1,** p. 1161; **Ref. 2,** p. 1697)

17. (D) Intestinal atresia and stenosis require surgical treatment but are not emergent. If midgut volvulus is not treated promptly, the intestine infarcts, resulting in severe short bowel syndrome. (**Ref. 1,** p. 1161; **Ref. 2,** pp. 1697–1698)

18. (C) Hypothermia, gastric distention, hypovolemia, and sepsis are preventible causes of morbidity in infants with abdominal wall defects. If the abdominal cavity is too small for primary repair, closure is staged with a silastic silo. (**Ref. 1,** pp. 1162–1163; **Ref. 2,** pp. 1706–1709)

19. (B) Diaphragmatic hernia usually occurs on the left side. Respiratory distress increases as the infant swallows air. Early diagnosis and extracorporeal membrane oxygenation (ECMO) have improved outcome but do not salvage infants with severe pulmonary hypoplasia. (**Ref. 1,** pp. 1163–1164; **Ref. 2,** p. 1686)

20. (A) Pyloric stenosis occurs proximal to the ampulla of Vater, so vomitus is nonbilious. All other obstructions are distal to the ampulla. (**Ref. 1,** p. 1165; **Ref. 2,** pp. 1694–1695)

21. **(E)** Both are defects of intrauterine closure of the abdominal wall, diagnosed in utero by ultrasound, and require surgical repair. Gastroschisis is always associated with nonrotation; most infants with omphalocele are malrotated. (**Ref. 1**, p. 1162; **Ref. 2**, pp. 1706–1709)

22. **(C)** Neonates require 120 calories per kg per day for growth. (**Ref. 1**, pp. 137, 1151)

23. **(D)** Instances of high alimentary tract obstruction associated with maternal polyhydramnios include esophageal atresia without tracheoesophageal fistula, pyloric atresia, duodenal atresia, and high jejunal atresia. Distal tracheoesophageal fistula with esophageal atresia permits passage of amniotic fluid into the intestinal tract. (**Ref. 1**, p. 1151)

24. **(B)** Colonic atresia is relatively uncommon and more often on the right than on the left. It is usually seen in full term infants. (**Ref. 1**, p. 1153)

25. **(A)** Internal drainage procedures such as cystoduodenostomy and cystojejunostomy are no longer recommended for choledochal cyst. The operation of choice is complete resection of the cyst and Roux-en-Y hepatojejunostomy. (**Ref. 1**, p. 1172; **Ref. 2**, pp. 1388, 1705)

26. **(E)** Children with neurologic impairment are the largest population with reflux. Bronchodilators reduce lower esophageal pressure. Esophageal atresia and diaphragmatic hernia affect the gastroesophageal angle. Reflux is one etiology for sudden infant death syndrome. (**Ref. 1**, p. 1166; **Ref. 2**, p. 1694)

27. **(D)** Gastroesophageal reflux may present with all listed symptoms except polyhydramnios. Most, but not all, patients vomit when they reflux. (**Ref. 1**, p. 1166; **Ref. 2**, p. 1694)

28. **(C)** Figure 13.1 shows two barium enema views of an ileocolic intussusception. This process in children is usually idiopathic and is most frequent in male toddlers. It causes small bowel obstruction and is often reduced in the radiology suite by careful contrast enema. A pathologic leadpoint (abnormality of the bowel wall) is

more common in males over 6 years of age and adults with intussusception. (**Ref. 1,** pp. 1167–1168; **Ref. 2,** p. 1700)

29. (B)   Nonhealing of the umbilical stump and omphalomesenteric and allantoic remnants are all causes for umbilical drainage. The mucosa of a Meckel's diverticulum does not connect to skin level. (**Ref. 1,** p. 1168; **Ref. 2,** pp. 1706–1708)

30. (A)   Ectopic gastric mucosa in Meckel's diverticulum takes up technetium–pertechnetate (as does a normal stomach) and may produce peptic ulceration. Pretreatment with pentagastrin and cimetidine improves scan results. (**Ref. 1,** p. 1169; **Ref. 2,** pp. 1701–1702)

31. (E)   Juvenile polyps are benign inflammatory lesions presenting between 4 and 14 years of age. Diagnosis is by endoscopy and air contrast barium enema. Symptomatic polyps are removed endoscopically. (**Ref. 1,** p. 1170; **Ref. 2,** pp. 1266–1267)

32. (D)   Biliary atresia presents with persistent neonatal jaundice without a mass. Early evaluation with surgery by 2 months of age markedly improves the success of portoenterostomy. Liver transplantation salvages infants with delayed diagnosis and failed drainage procedures. (**Ref. 1,** p. 1171; **Ref. 2,** p. 1704)

33. (C)   All listed tests are appropriate in the work-up of neonatal jaundice. If biliary atresia is suspected, early operative exploration markedly improves the success of a drainage procedure. (**Ref. 1,** p. 1171; **Ref. 2,** p. 1704)

34. (B)   A young child gives no history, so physical examination is the key to diagnosis. Delay in diagnosis is common, increasing the incidence of dehydration, gangrene, and perforation. Incidental appendectomy is performed by inversion. (**Ref. 1,** p. 1173)

35. (A)   There is a large differential diagnosis for acute abdominal pain in children, including all those listed except acute renal failure. Meckel's diverticulitis requires surgery, but the rest are usually managed medically. (**Ref. 1,** p. 1173)

36. (E) Appendicitis is usually associated with dehydration and ketosis. If the appendix is near the ureter or bladder, there may be a few red and/or white cells. Many bacteria signal a urinary tract infection or contaminated specimen. (**Ref. 1,** p. 1173)

37. (D) Capillary hemangiomas are much more common than cavernous. All other statements are correct. (**Ref. 5,** pp. 77–78)

38. (C) Suppurative cervical lymphadenitis is often caused by *Staphylococcus,* and antibiotic therapy must cover this organism. The other organisms are less common causes of cervical lymph gland enlargement. (**Ref. 1,** p. 1176)

39. (B) Neck masses in young children are rarely malignant. Infection and benign congenital remnants are most frequent. (**Ref. 1,** p. 1176)

40. (A) Inguinal hernias incarcerate most frequently in infants. Hernias in premature infants should be repaired prior to initial hospital discharge, and other infant hernias should be repaired soon after diagnosis. Delay in repair is not warranted. (**Ref. 1,** p. 1176)

41. (E) Ovaries are the most common structure to enter a female hernia sac. The ovary frequently incarcerates but, in contrast to the male testis and small bowel, rarely infarcts. All other answers are correct. (**Ref. 2,** p. 1711; **Ref. 5,** pp. 69–70)

42. (E) Most cryptorchid testes are unilateral, palpable, associated with a hernia sac, and at risk for torsion. The incidence of malignancy is much higher than in descended testes, and orchiopexy secures the testis where it can be observed. (**Ref. 2,** p. 1711; **Ref. 5,** pp. 71–72)

43. (C) Orchiopexy is ideally performed soon after the first birthday. This permits time for spontaneous descent to occur. (**Ref. 1,** p. 1178; **Ref. 2,** p. 1712)

44. (B) Umbilical hernias with fascial defects greater than 2 cm usually do not close spontaneously. All other statements are correct. (**Ref. 1,** p. 1178; **Ref. 2,** p. 1707)

45. (E)   Chest x-ray following aspiration of a foreign body is helpful only if there are positive findings. Atelectasis, mediastinal shift, and air trapping may suggest the presence of a bronchial obstruction caused by the foreign body, but these may not be present. If the history is strongly suggestive, bronchoscopy is indicated even if the x-ray is normal. (**Ref. 2,** pp. 1689–1690; **Ref. 5,** pp. 84–85)

46. (D)   Most esophageal foreign bodies pass spontaneously. Button batteries contain mercuric oxide, which can leak and cause esophageal perforation. Blunt foreign bodies can be removed under fluoroscopy with a balloon catheter. Sharp objects require endoscopic removal. (**Ref. 2,** pp. 1689–1690; **Ref. 5,** p. 85)

47. (C)   All medical personnel are mandated reporters of suspected child abuse. Determination of abuse and abuser is left to the appropriate government agency. (**Ref. 5,** p. 83)

48. (B)   Epigastric and perineal trauma, long bone fractures in young children, and all burns are suspicious for child abuse or neglect. Solid organ trauma more commonly follows blunt accidental trauma. (**Ref. 5,** p. 83)

49. (A)   The leading cause of death in children is accidental injury. Malignancies are the second most frequent cause of pediatric mortality. (**Ref. 1,** p. 1174)

50. (E)   The primary mechanism of injury for pediatric trauma is blunt rather than penetrating. All other statements are correct. (**Ref. 1,** p. 1174)

51. (D)   Rapid volume expansion with isotonic fluids (20 cc/kg) restores vital signs in most hypovolemic injured children. Vascular access and adequate gas exchange are also important. Vasopressors are rarely indicated. (**Ref. 1,** p. 1175; **Ref. 2,** pp. 1682–1683)

52. (C)   Diagnostic peritoneal lavage is infrequently performed in children. Solid organ injury with hemoperitoneum is not an indication for surgery unless vital signs fail to stabilize with crystalloid resuscitation. (**Ref. 1,** p. 1175)

53. **(E)** Histology is the major determinant of survival in patients with Wilms' tumor. All other statements are correct. (**Ref. 1,** pp. 1179–1180; **Ref. 2,** p. 1714)

54. **(D)** Most children with neuroblastoma have advanced disease at the time of diagnosis. Age at diagnosis is the other determinant of survival. All other statements are correct. (**Ref. 1,** pp. 1180–1181; **Ref. 2,** pp. 1714–1715)

55. **(C)** Wilms' tumor and neuroblastoma are the two most frequent abdominal tumors in infants and young children. (**Ref. 1,** pp. 1179–1180; **Ref. 2,** p. 1714)

56. **(B)** Sacrococcygeal teratoma is much more common in females than in males. Most are benign at birth, but the incidence of malignancy increases rapidly with age. All other statements are correct. (**Ref. 1,** p. 1183; **Ref. 2,** p. 1716)

57. **(E)** The history is classic for hypertrophic pyloric stenosis. Gastroesophageal reflux is the primary differential diagnosis. Duodenal stenosis, adrenogenital syndrome, and aminoaciduria are rare. (**Ref. 1,** p. 1166; **Ref. 2,** pp. 1694–1695)

58. **(D)** The hypertrophied pylorus is palpable in the epigastrium of a quiet infant with an empty stomach. Gastric contractions may be visible in the upper abdomen. There is no abdominal distention or tenderness, and bowel sounds are normal. (**Ref. 1,** p. 1165; **Ref. 2,** pp. 1694–1695)

59. **(C)** In the rare case where the "olive" is nonpalpable, a hypertrophic pylorus can usually be identified by ultrasound examination (see Figure 13.2), which shows longitudinal and cross-section images of an elongated pyloric channel with thickened musculature. This finding is called a "target" sign. If ultrasound is not diagnostic, and the infant continues to vomit, an upper gastrointestinal (UGI) series is obtained. (**Ref. 1,** p. 1165; **Ref. 2,** p. 1695)

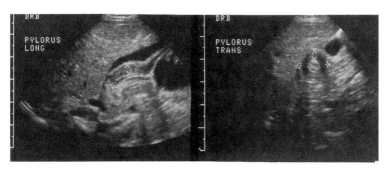

Figure 13.2

60. (B) The triad of abdominal colic, vomiting, and currant-jelly stools in a child immediately raises the suspicion of intussusception. The other diagnoses are not associated with pain, and most do not occur at this age. (**Ref. 1,** p. 1167; **Ref. 2,** p. 1700)

61. (A) The ileocolic leadpoint produces distal intestinal obstruction with increased bowel sounds. The mass moves around the colon, occasionally as far as the rectum. (**Ref. 1,** p. 1167)

62. (E) Absence of cecal gas in the right lower quadrant is consistent with intussusception. Dilated loops of distal small bowel may also be present, indicating the obstructive nature of the intussusception. (**Ref. 1,** p. 1167; **Ref. 2,** p. 1700)

63. (D) A contrast enema is diagnostic, and often therapeutic, for ileocolic intussusception. The retrograde barium column may both diagnose and reverse the intussusception. Care must be taken to rule out any sign of peritonitis (fever, leukocytosis, diffuse tenderness, rigidity) before attempts at enema reduction. (**Ref. 1,** p. 1168; **Ref. 2,** p. 1701)

64. (E) The above findings are most consistent with an incarcerated inguinal hernia. Hydroceles present in the scrotum. (**Ref. 1,** p. 1177; **Ref. 2,** pp. 1710–1711)

65. (A)   It is often possible to safely reduce an incarcerated hernia in infants and convert an emergency that requires immediate operation to an elective procedure. Incision and drainage and needle aspiration are not indicated. Intravenous antibiotics have no place as sole treatment, and duplex ultrasound is not likely to help. (**Ref. 1,** p. 1177; **Ref. 2,** p. 1711)

66. (C)   Unlike undescended testicles, incarcerated hernias are not associated with infertility. (**Ref. 1,** p. 1177; **Ref. 2,** p. 1711)

14

Case Studies

DIRECTIONS (Questions 1 through 28): This section consists of a clinical situation followed by a series of questions. Study the situation and select the ONE best answer to each question following it.

Questions 1 through 3

A 22-year-old student is seen in the emergency room with a complaint of increasing right lower quadrant abdominal pain. He awoke 6 hours earlier with vague central abdominal pain. He tried to return to sleep, but could not due to discomfort. He has never had similar pain. He is not hungry and is mildly nauseated. Past medical history is unremarkable. Physical exam reveals point tenderness in the right lower quadrant, depressed bowel sounds, pain referred to the right with pressure in the left lower quadrant. Rectal exam is unremarkable; stool occult blood test is negative. White blood cell count is 12,300, urinalysis is normal, and he is afebrile.

  1. The MOST likely diagnosis is
    A. diverticulitis
    B. acute appendicitis
    C. ureterolithiasis
    D. cholecystitis
    E. abdominal aortic aneurysm (AAA)

2. Treatment of the above patient should be
  A. intravenous antibiotics only
  B. intravenous fluids only
  C. IV fluid, IV antibiotics, operation
  D. clinic follow-up if symptoms do not subside
  E. arteriogram

3. The treatment goal in operating for appendicitis is
  A. operate only on patients when the diagnosis of appendicitis is certain
  B. operate on anyone with right lower quadrant pain
  C. accept a few ruptured appendices in order to prevent negative operations
  D. operate upon unexplained right lower quadrant pain in otherwise acceptable operative candidates
  E. remove the appendix at every possible chance during other abdominal operations

Questions 4 and 5

A 2.5-cm nodule is found on physical exam in the right lobe of the thyroid in a 35-year-old woman. She is asymptomatic and has no clinical evidence of overt hyperthyroidism.

4. Further evaluation may include all of the following EXCEPT
  A. measurement of serum T_3
  B. measurement of serum T_4
  C. measurement of serum thyroid-stimulating hormone (TSH)
  D. reassurance only
  E. fine-needle aspiration cytology

5. The nodule is found to be nonfunctioning on thyroid scan, and a needle aspiration biopsy is interpreted as a "follicular neoplasm." The NEXT step in caring for this patient would be to
   A. reassure the patient and reexamine with ultrasound in 6 months
   B. begin suppression therapy with L-thyroxine to shrink the nodule
   C. perform an incisional biopsy of the nodule in the operating room
   D. remove the right lobe and isthmus of this patient's thyroid
   E. perform a total thyroidectomy and right-sided modified radical lymph node dissection

Questions 6 through 8

A 54-year-old alcoholic male presents to the emergency center with a 2-day history of severe epigastric pain and nausea and vomiting. He is afebrile with tenderness over his epigastrium. There is voluntary guarding present. The pain is more severe on lying supine and radiates through to the central back.

6. Appropriate tests to perform to further evaluate this patient include all of the following EXCEPT
   A. abdominal x-ray series
   B. ultrasound of the abdomen
   C. heme profile
   D. upper gastrointestinal endoscopy following 6 weeks of antacid therapy
   E. serum amylase and lipase

7. His abdominal series shows no free air. His ultrasound shows no gallstones, but the pancreas is enlarged. The common bile duct is mildly dilated. Serum amylase and lipase are markedly elevated. His Pao_2 on 2 L/min nasal oxygen is 50 mm Hg. A reasonable working diagnosis at this point would be
   A. peptic ulcer disease
   B. cholecystitis
   C. pancreatitis
   D. ruptured abdominal aortic aneurysm
   E. diverticulitis

8. You wish to be able to get some idea of how severe this episode is. All of the following data is related to severity prediction EXCEPT
   A. amylase
   B. hematocrit change
   C. arterial blood gas
   D. amount of intravenous fluid required
   E. blood glucose

Questions 9 and 11

A 50-year-old man presented to his personal physician with the complaint of morning headaches that had progressively worsened over the past 2 months. A magnetic resonance image (MRI) scan revealed an extensive, unresectable mass lesion suggestive of a primary brain tumor.

9. All of the following are true about intracranial gliomas EXCEPT
   A. they are the most common intracranial tumor in adults
   B. they rarely undergo malignant degeneration
   C. they almost never metastasize to other organs
   D. permanent cure is unlikely
   E. they typically arise in the cerebral hemispheres in adults

10. Another common presentation of brain tumors in adults is
   A. recent weight gain
   B. loss of recent memory
   C. new onset seizure disorder
   D. high-frequency hearing loss
   E. anorexia

11. It is decided to treat the patient with radiation therapy. In preparation for this, the patient is given glucocorticoid therapy. The purpose of this pretreatment is to
   A. improve the cure rate of the radiation therapy
   B. decrease brain swelling
   C. prevent hair loss
   D. prevent memory loss
   E. help shrink the tumor

Question 12 through 16

The mother of a 6-year-old girl calls your office because the child has abdominal pain and vomiting.

12. Relevant questions include all of the following EXCEPT
    A. duration of pain
    B. insurance status
    C. temperature
    D. time of last void
    E. location of pain

13. The pain started 24 hours ago, and the child won't say where it hurts most. She feels hot, is anorectic, and can't remember when she last voided. You recommend
    A. close parental observation at home
    B. admission for IV hydration
    C. oral antibiotics
    D. clear liquids and acetaminophen
    E. surgical consultation

14. Which of the following physical exam findings does NOT help distinguish a surgical from a nonsurgical abdominal problem?
    A. dry mucous membranes
    B. limited patient movement
    C. absent bowel sounds
    D. abdominal tenderness
    E. rectal tenderness

15. Initial work-up includes all of the following EXCEPT
    A. complete blood count (CBC)
    B. urinalysis
    C. serum electrolytes
    D. liver function tests
    E. abdominal x-rays

16. Appropriate management includes all of the following EXCEPT
    A. lactated Ringer's bolus
    B. pelvic examination
    C. nasogastric sump

D. operative exploration
E. intravenous antibiotics

Questions 17 through 24

A 25-year-old patient is brought to the emergency room following a motorcycle accident. His blood pressure is 80/60 mm Hg; pulse 160 beats/min; respiratory rate, 40 breaths/min, labored. He has an obvious open left femur fracture and is complaining vigorously of left chest pain and inability to get his breath. He refuses to lie flat.

17. Initial assessment would include all of the following EXCEPT
A. auscultation of both lung fields
B. palpation of the position of the trachea
C. sending the patient for chest x-ray
D. looking to see if neck veins are distended
E. cardiac auscultation

18. His neck veins are found to be distended, trachea is shifted to the right, and there are absent breath sounds on the left. He is becoming more agitated and is demanding that someone help him breathe. Appropriate action would be to
A. order a stat chest x-ray
B. paralyze and intubate the patient
C. place a left chest tube
D. perform a nasotracheal intubation
E. place a needle in the second left intercostal space in the midclavicular line

19. Appropriate treatment was performed, and the patient is breathing easier now. His BP is 80/60; pulse, 140; and respiratory rate, 35. His breath sounds are equal bilaterally and his neck veins are flat. Initial treatment of his shock would include all of the following EXCEPT
A. transfusion of uncrossmatched blood
B. starting two large bore IVs
C. infusing two liters of Ringer's lactate as rapidly as possible
D. controlling any external hemorrhage
E. placing him on high-flow oxygen

20. After infusion of two L Ringer's lactate over ten minutes, his vital signs are unchanged. His neck veins remain flat and he is oliguric. How much intravascular volume may you assume he has lost?
  A. <10%
  B. >35%
  C. about 500 mL of blood
  D. about 750 mL of blood
  E. <30%

21. Your treatment of his hypotension now would be to
  A. order a computed tomography (CT) scan of his abdomen
  B. continue transfusion of crystalloid and order O-negative or type-specific blood for immediate transfusion
  C. continue transfusion of crystalloid only
  D. start dopamine infusion
  E. order blood transfusion as soon as fully typed and cross-matched blood is available

22. Appropriate initial treatment of his hypotension has been carried out. His blood pressure is now 130/90; pulse, 100; and respiration, 25. External hemorrhage is controlled; neck veins are flat. Chest x-ray shows no evidence of hemorrhage, and chest tube drainage is minimal. He is beginning to complain of left upper quadrant pain and is requiring an IV rate of 300 mL/hr to prevent hypotension from recurring. Considerations regarding reasons for recurring hypotension include all of the following EXCEPT
  A. intraperitoneal source of bleeding
  B. continued bleeding at femur fracture site
  C. pericardial tamponade
  D. possible pelvic fracture as source of bleeding
  E. inadequate initial volume replacement

23. In view of the above, all of the following would be appropriate actions EXCEPT
  A. diagnostic peritoneal lavage
  B. x-ray of the pelvis
  C. monitoring of urine output
  D. placement of central venous line for monitoring
  E. pericardiocentesis

24. X-ray of his pelvis shows no fracture. His vital signs are now normal and stable. He continues to complain of increasing left upper quadrant pain. The orthopaedic surgeon wishes to take this patient to the operating room to fix his open femur fracture. You should

A. transfer care of this patient to the orthopaedic surgeon

B. exclude an intraperitoneal source of hemorrhage by diagnostic peritoneal lavage (DPL) or CT scan

C. order a tagged red cell scan

D. admit the patient for 3 days of observation before treatment of his fracture

E. ask the orthopaedic surgeon to do the operation under local anesthesia

Questions 25 through 28

A middle-aged male with known hypertension suddenly experiences excruciating pain in his back between the shoulder blades. The pain does not radiate to the neck or arm. Examination reveals a systolic murmur over the aortic area radiating to the major vessels. There is a difference in the blood pressure in the two arms.

25. The probable clinical diagnosis is

A. myocardial infarction

B. angina pectoris

C. coarctation of the aorta

D. acute disk prolapse

E. dissecting aneurysm

26. The most useful initial test would be

A. electrocardiogram (ECG)

B. stress test and ECG

C. esophogram

D. x-ray of the thoracic spine

E. x-ray of the chest

27. The important finding on the above examination would be
   A. Q waves
   B. sagging of the ST segment
   C. narrowing of the lower end of the esophagus
   D. narrowing of the intervertebral space
   E. widening of the mediastinum, aortic wall calcification, and left pleural effusion

28. The ideal treatment would be
   A. sedation, O_2, and digoxin
   B. aortocoronary bypass grafting
   C. antacids
   D. laminectomy
   E. reduction of hypertension; if this fails, then operation

---

DIRECTIONS (Questions 29 and 30): Each of the questions or incomplete statements below is followed by five answers or completions. Select the ONE that is best in each case.

---

29. A 62-year-old black male with a positive family history of prostate cancer comes in for his yearly physical exam. He is found to have a prostatic nodule that was not felt last year. The most reliable method of diagnosing (or excluding) prostatic carcinoma is
   A. prostatic acid phosphatase
   B. prostatic specific antigen (PSA)
   C. transrectal biopsy
   D. prostate ultrasound
   E. radionuclide bone scan

30. All of the following are acceptable therapeutic options for asymptomatic metastatic prostatic carcinoma EXCEPT
   A. observation
   B. testosterone
   C. orchiectomy
   D. estrogens
   E. luteinizing hormone-releasing hormone (LHRH) analogs

Case Studies

Answers and Comments

1. (B) This case illustrates classical presentation of acute appendicitis. Diverticulitis and AAA are unlikely in this age group. The pain is not the correct character for urolithiasis nor the correct location for cholecystitis. (**Ref. 6,** p. 443)

2. (C) This patient should undergo prompt appendectomy. Waiting for any significant period only increases the risk of perforation. Antibiotic therapy alone is not indicated for a diagnosis of appendicitis in a reasonable operative candidate. (**Ref. 6,** pp. 450–451)

3. (D) A patient who presents with diffuse abdominal pain becoming well localized to the right lower quadrant, *and* whose pain symptoms may not adequately be explained by some other likely process, *and* who is able to readily withstand the stress of operation, should be operated upon with a presumed diagnosis of appendicitis. This approach will allow early diagnosis and treatment when the process does not pose a significant threat of peritonitis. (**Ref. 1,** pp. 885–891)

4. (D) Reassurance only is not appropriate in the evaluation of this patient. All other options are reasonable in evaluation of this thyroid nodule. (**Ref. 1,** pp. 582–584)

5. **(D)** Fine-needle aspiration cannot distinguish between benign and malignant follicular neoplasms; if the tumor proves to be a malignancy on frozen section following a thyroid lobectomy and isthmusectomy, the surgeon should proceed with a total or near-total thyroidectomy and a lymph node dissection if clinically indicated. (**Ref. 1,** p. 584; **Ref. 2,** pp. 1632–1633)

6. **(D)** While peptic ulcer disease cannot be excluded without further study, presumptive treatment and 6-week follow-up is not warranted in this acute presentation. An abdominal series would be reasonable to exclude free intraperitoneal air; an ultrasound and amylase and lipase to screen for hepatobiliary disease; and a heme profile to evaluate hemoglobin level and white blood cell count. (**Ref. 1,** pp. 736–746)

7. **(A)** While a posterior penetrating peptic ulcer cannot be totally excluded, pancreatitis is most likely. Cholecystitis should have more definite findings of wall thickness and pericholecystic fluid to be considered. Pancreatitis fits the pain presentation and ultrasound report and is supported by elevated amylase and lipase values. Pulmonary dysfunction may also accompany pancreatitis. (**Ref. 1,** pp. 1081–1082)

8. **(A)** Hemoconcentration of 10%, hypoxia (PaO_2 <60 mm Hg), hyperglycemia (blood sugar >200 mg/dL), and amount of intravenous fluid required over the first 24 hours of hospitalization, have a bearing on prognosis; the level of the serum amylase value does not. (**Ref. 1,** p. 1084; **Ref. 6,** p. 574)

9. **(B)** Glial tumors are usually found above the tentorium (i.e., in the cerebral hemispheres). They rarely metastasize and permanent cure is unlikely. They are frequently poorly differentiated and undergo malignant degeneration. (**Ref. 5,** p. 312)

10. **(C)** New-onset seizure disorder in adults suggests brain tumor. This presumed diagnosis must be excluded by appropriate imaging studies. The other choices are more rarely associated with intracranial neoplasm. (**Ref. 3,** p. 1861)

11. **(B)** It is well established that steroid pretreatment helps decrease brain swelling induced by radiation therapy. The therapy must be started before the radiation. (**Ref. 6,** p. 834)

12. **(B)** A careful, detailed history is important to establish the exact time of onset, duration and location of pain, and patient hydration status. (**Ref. 1,** p. 1173)

13. **(E)** The child's symptoms are suggestive of an acute abdomen with significant dehydration, requiring hospitalization and surgical consultation. (**Ref. 1,** p. 1173)

14. **(A)** Dry mucous membranes are associated with dehydration, which can occur with either surgical or nonsurgical problems. All other signs are suggestive of peritonitis. (**Ref. 1,** p. 1173)

15. **(D)** Laboratory evaluation for appendicitis includes CBC and urinalysis. If the patient appears severely dehydrated, serum electrolytes should be obtained. Abdominal x-ray should be obtained and may reveal a calcified appendicolith. (**Ref. 1,** p. 1173)

16. **(B)** Since this patient is significantly dehydrated, an intravenous fluid bolus is necessary to stabilize the patient prior to an operative procedure. Nasogastric catheter and intravenous antibiotics are also warranted. (**Ref. 1,** p. 1173)

17. **(C)** The patient is in severe respiratory distress. Sending him for any study is not indicated until his condition can be stabilized. (**Ref. 1,** p. 260)

18. **(E)** All findings presented are consistent with the presence of a left-sided tension pneumothorax. Urgent treatment, which entails immediate needle thoracentesis, is required, followed by chest tube insertion. (**Ref. 1,** p. 262)

19. **(A)** The patient has received no prior fluid resuscitation as of yet. While uncrossmatched blood may eventually be indicated, vigorous crystalloid fluid infusion is appropriate at this point. (**Ref. 1,** p. 39)

20. (B) Significant blood loss is indicated by lack of response to rapid fluid infusion. The patient demonstrates evidence of hypovolemic shock. (**Ref. 1,** p. 37)

21. (B) Uncrossmatched blood is now indicated, but crystalloid infusion should be continued, pending the availability of blood. (**Ref. 1,** pp. 39–40)

22. (C) In a patient with flat neck veins who is now hypotensive, pericardial tamponade is unlikely. There is nothing in his examination to suggest this diagnosis. (**Ref. 1,** p. 43)

23. (E) Again, there is low probability for tamponade. Pericardiocentesis is not indicated in this situation. (**Ref. 1,** p. 43)

24. (B) Prior to repair of the orthopaedic injury in the operating room, where the patient's physical exam cannot be monitored (due to anesthesia), a suspected source of intra-abdominal injury should be rapidly excluded by either DPL or CT scan. Local anesthesia is not an option for repair of the femur fracture. (**Ref. 1,** p. 266)

25. (E) The sudden onset of excruciating pain in the back in a hypertensive individual should lead one to suspect an acute dissecting aneurysm. The presence of a systolic murmur is a further suggestion of this process. The proximal extent of the dissection probably involves the left subclavian origin and, hence, the difference in the blood pressure reading between the two arms. (**Ref. 2,** p. 916)

26. (E) X-ray of the chest would be the most useful initial examination; it shows dilatation of the aortic shadow. (**Ref. 2,** p. 917)

27. (E) Examination would show widening of the mediastinum, calcification of the aortic wall, and possibly a left pleural effusion. If the aneurysm ruptures into the left pleural cavity, this effusion may be blood. (**Ref. 2,** p. 917)

28. (E) The initial treatment of dissecting aneurysm is that of reducing the blood pressure and rate of ejection of blood from the left ventricle. If this does not improve the situation or the dissection continues, surgery is required. Operative treatments include fenestration to return the blood from the false passage into the lumen or replacement of the diseased artery by a Dacron prosthesis. (**Ref. 2,** p. 917)

29. **(C)**   Transrectal, or any other biopsy which produces tissue, is the best means of diagnosing malignancy. PSA is used for screening, as evidence for or against metastasis, and for surveillance of metastatic disease. It is not as accurate as tissue diagnosis. Other choices provide indirect evidence of benign or malignant disease. (**Ref. 5,** p. 347)

30. **(B)**   The androgen dependency of most prostatic tumors was recognized more than 50 years ago. A marked therapeutic response is frequently observed with androgen ablation in the form of orchiectomy or estrogen or antiandrogen administration. Observation of asymptomatic patients is reasonable because of the slow-growing nature of these tumors. (**Ref. 5,** p. 349)